ANNUAL REVIEW of NURSING EDUCATION

Volume 5, 2007

Challenges and New Directions in Nursing Education

Marilyn H. Oermann, PhD, RN, FAAN, Editor
Kathleen T. Heinrich, PhD, RN, Associate Editor

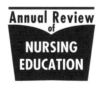

Annual Review
of
NURSING
EDUCATION

SPRINGER PUBLISHING COMPANY
New York

To purchase copies of other volumes of the *Annual Review of Nursing Education* at 10% off the list price, go to www.springerpub.com/ARNE.

Springer Publishing Company, LLC
11 West 42nd Street, 15th Floor
New York, NY 10036-8002
www.springerpub.com

07 08 09 10/5 4 3 2 1

ISBN-0-8261-02395
ISSN-1542-412X

ANNUAL REVIEW OF NURSING EDUCATION is indexed in *Cumulative Index to Nursing* and *Allied Health Literature*.

Printed in the United States of America by Bang Printing.

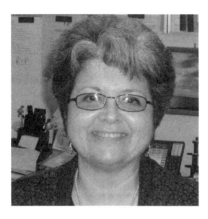

This volume is dedicated to the memory of Jo-Ann L. Rossitto, DNSc, RN (1951–2006) who served as an editorial board member for the Annual Review of Nursing Education (ARNE) *since its inception. Energetic, loyal, and committed, Jo-Ann's support for the scholarship of teaching and learning extended far beyond her ARNE responsibilities. The Dean and Director of Nursing Education at San Diego City College, Jo-Ann inspired student and faculty colleagues to pursue educational and professional opportunities. While our scholarly pursuits were enriched by Jo-Ann's generosity in life, her legacy is a challenge to educate, lead, and mentor nurse-scholars by example.*

Contents

**Part III: Enhancing Learning and Student Development
Through Technology and Assessment**

Contributors

Mary-Anne Andrusyszyn, EdD, RN
Associate Professor
School of Nursing
Faculty of Health Sciences
University of Western Ontario
London, Ontario, Canada

Lenore Bertone, BS, RN
Nurse Therapist
South Beach Psychiatric Center
Staten Island, New York

Charlene Beynon, MScN, RN
Director
Research Education Evaluation &
  Development Services
Middlesex-London Health Unit
London, Ontario, Canada

Diane M. Billings, EdD, RN, FAAN
Chancellor's Professor of Nursing
Indiana University School of
  Nursing
Indianapolis, Indiana

John B. Blyth, MBA, MIS
Education Specialist and Web
  Developer
School of Nursing
University at Buffalo, The State
  University of New York
Buffalo, New York

Richard Booth, MScN(c), RN
Research Assistant
School of Nursing
Faculty of Health Sciences
University of Western Ontario
London, Ontario, Canada

Jo-Ann Douglas, BS, RN
Staff Nurse
Beth Israel Medical Center
New York, New York

W. Scott Erdley, DNS, RN
Clinical Associate Professor
School of Nursing
University at Buffalo, The State
  University of New York
Buffalo, New York

Linda Felver, PhD, RN
Associate Professor and Director,
    Older Adult Focus Project
School of Nursing
Oregon Health & Science
    University
Portland, Oregon

Nel Glass, PhD, MHPEd, BA,
    Dip Neuroscience Nursing,
    RN, FCN(NSW),
    FRCNA
Associate Professor
Department of Nursing and
    Health Care Practices
School of Health and Human
    Sciences
Southern Cross University
Lismore, Australia

Dolly Goldenberg, PhD, RN
Professor and Chair of Graduate
    Programs
School of Nursing
Faculty of Health Sciences
University of Western Ontario
London, Ontario, Canada

Linda M. Goodfellow, PhD, RN
Associate Professor
Duquesne University School of
    Nursing
Pittsburgh, Pennsylvania

Carroll L. Iwasiw, EdD, RN
Professor
School of Nursing
Faculty of Health Sciences
University of Western Ontario
London, Ontario, Canada

Marianne R. Jeffreys, EdD, RN
Professor, Nursing
Nursing Department
The City University of New York
    College of Staten Island
Staten Island, New York

Louise Sherman Jenkins, PhD,
    RN
Co-Director, Clinical Education
    and Evaluation Laboratory
Co-Director, Institute for
    Educators in Nursing and
    Health Professions
School of Nursing
University of Maryland
Baltimore, Maryland

Janice M. Jones, PhD, RN, CNS
Clinical Associate Professor
School of Nursing
University at Buffalo, The State
    University of New York
Buffalo, New York

Jayne Kendle, MS(N), RNC
Associate Professor
Department of Nursing
Saint Mary's College
Notre Dame, Indiana

Jill Laroussini, MSN, RN
Instructor, College of Nursing and
    Allied Health
University of Louisiana at
    Lafayette
Lafayette, Louisiana

Gwen Leigh, MSN, RN
Instructor, College of Nursing and
  Allied Health
University of Louisiana at
  Lafayette
Lafayette, Louisiana

**Kristen Lethbridge, MScN, RN,
  PhD(c)**
Research Coordinator
School of Nursing
Faculty of Health Sciences
University of Western Ontario
London, Ontario, Canada

Vivien Li, BS, RN
Staff Nurse
Lutheran Medical Center
Brooklyn, New York

**Susan Luparell, PhD, APRN,
  BC**
Assistant Professor
College of Nursing
Montana State
  University–Bozeman
Great Falls Campus
Great Falls, Montana

Gene Majka, MS, RN
Instructor
Barry University School of
  Nursing
Miami Shores, Florida

Cathy Mawdsley, MScN, RN
Clinical Nurse Specialist – Critical
  Care
University Hospital
London, Ontario, Canada

Ruth Neese, MSN, RN, CEN
Adjunct Faculty
Palm Beach Community College –
  Eissey Campus
Palm Beach Gardens, Florida

**Ramona Nelson, PhD, RN,
  FAAN**
Professor and Chair
Department of Nursing
Slippery Rock University
Slippery Rock, Pennsylvania

Sara Newman, BS, RN
Staff Nurse
Beth Israel Medical Center
New York, New York

Cathy Parsons, MScN, RN
Nursing Practice Consultant/
  Corporate Facilitator
St. Joseph's Health Care London
London, Ontario, Canada

Sudha C. Patel, DNS, RN, MA
Assistant Professor, College of
  Nursing and Allied Health
University of Louisiana at
  Lafayette
Lafayette, Louisiana

Paulette Demaske Rollant, PhD, RN
President, Rollant Concepts, Inc.
Test-Prep/Curriculum Specialist
Navarre Beach, Florida

Kay Sackett, EdD, RN
Clinical Associate Professor
School of Nursing
University at Buffalo, The State
    University of New York
Buffalo, New York

Kathy Schaivone, MPA
Managing Director, Clinical
    Education and Evaluation
    Laboratory
Schools of Nursing and Medicine
University of Maryland
Baltimore, Maryland

Barbara Sinclair, MScN, RN
Coordinator for Simulated
    Clinical Education
School of Nursing
Faculty of Health Sciences
University of Western Ontario
London, Ontario, Canada

Ardith L. Sudduth, PhD, RN, MA, APRN-BC
Assistant Professor, College of
    Nursing and Allied Health
University of Louisiana at
    Lafayette
Lafayette, Louisiana

Geneiva G. Tennant, MSN, RN
Charge Nurse
North Shore Medical Center
Miami, Florida

Catherine Van Son, PhD, RN
Postdoctoral Fellow and
    Instructor
School of Nursing
Oregon Health & Science
    University
Portland, Oregon

Linda H. Zoeller, PhD, APRN, BC
Chair and Associate Professor
Department of Nursing
Saint Mary's College
Notre Dame, Indiana

Preface

When we first envisioned the *Annual Review of Nursing Education* (ARNE), our intent was to gather each year's hottest trends and cutting edge innovations into one volume. In the process of editing this fifth volume, we noticed that these chapters are not only in the vanguard of nursing education, but they also reflect issues that are igniting national discourse. One of the ARNE chapters relates to an increase in academic incivility; the front page of *The New York Times* carried an article about legislation that has New York leading a "politeness trend" (Hu, 2006, p. 1). Other ARNE chapters describe the lessons nurse educators and students learned from surviving the Gulf Coast hurricanes and the implications of foreign nurses' immigration on American nursing education, thus reflecting national and international concerns expressed often in the media. Increasingly, nurse educators' insights and recommendations for turning teaching challenges into opportunities can serve as an inspiration for national and global action.

Part I of this year's ARNE focuses on clinical nursing education. Chapters explain how to use standardized patients for clinical teaching and evaluation, share two innovative clinical experiences for students, and present the findings of the first phase of a research study on a formal mentoring program for beginning nursing students.

Nurse educators face many challenges in selecting clinical sites, planning clinical learning activities, providing feedback to students, and evaluating their competencies. In chapter 1, Louise Sherman Jenkins and Kathy Schaivone explain how standardized patients can help educators overcome some of these barriers to effective clinical teaching and evaluation. This form of simulation allows learners to practice skills with a real person in a safe and controlled environment. Having simulated patients trained to portray focused scenarios provides for consistency of experiences across learners and strengthens the reliability of the evaluation process. The authors provide sufficient detail and many examples of using standardized patients in undergraduate and graduate courses for faculty to integrate this method in their own programs.

Nurse educators are challenged to provide innovative and meaningful educational opportunities to enhance the cultural competency of nursing students. Marianne R. Jeffreys, Lenore Bertone, Jo-Ann Douglas, Vivien Li, and Sara Newman, in chapter 2, describe a multidimensional strategy for learning and teaching cultural competence in graduate nursing education. The strategy involves an innovative field trip experience. The authors provide background information about the strategy development, implementation, and evaluation, including an empirically supported model to guide cultural competence education— the Cultural Competence and Confidence model. Four case exemplars demonstrate how this strategy is applied in clinical nursing education at the graduate level. The strategy also could be used with prelicensure students.

Faculty teaching in undergraduate nursing programs are continually challenged to find meaningful clinical experiences for their students. As student enrollments increase and patients' lengths of stays decrease, this challenge is becoming even more difficult. In chapter 3, Jayne Kendle and Linda Zoeller describe a service learning clinical experience. "Time Out" is a pediatric respite care experience in which nursing students provide respite care in the home for families with children who have special needs. The authors describe the benefits of this type of clinical experience for nursing students, guidelines for students and families, program evaluation, and outcomes of the program. Tools used to evaluate student learning are shared with readers.

Mentoring is a voluntary partnership in which an individual with knowledge and experience, a mentor, acts as a role model for a student or nurse with less experience over an extended period of time. Mentoring is a valuable component of a nursing student's education, but instruments for assessing the characteristics and outcomes of mentoring in nursing education are lacking. In chapter 4, Mary-Anne Andrusyszyn, Carroll L. Iwasiw, Dolly Goldenberg, and their research team of Cathy Mawdsley, Barbara Sinclair, Charlene Beynon, Cathy Parsons, Kristen Lethbridge, and Richard Booth describe the first phase of a 3-year research study on a formal mentoring program for beginning baccalaureate nursing students in Canada. The authors present how they developed and pilot tested questionnaires to assess the outcomes of this mentoring program and share the mentor pretest with readers.

Chapters in Part II of the *Annual Review* address some of the challenging aspects of teaching in nursing. We begin this part with a chapter by Susan Luparell on student incivility and dealing with rude, unprofessional, and inappropriate behaviors among nursing students. The purpose of her chapter is to share some of the mistakes she made and the lessons she learned in dealing with difficult or challenging student situations as a nurse educator. Strategies to prevent and address this type of incivility are suggested. A national survey of nursing faculty confirmed that educators are confronted with problematic student behaviors in astonishingly high numbers. Read this chapter before encountering these student behaviors in your own teaching.

Issues such as competitiveness, lack of support, and workplace violence affect academics' individual development and their ability to effectively take on new educational initiatives. In chapter 6, Nel Glass shares the experiences of women nurse academics who participated in a postmodern feminist, ethnographic study that involved four countries (Australia, New Zealand, the United Kingdom, and the United States) over an 8-year period (1997-2004). Dr. Glass explores the competitive university cultures and the hope and optimism nurse academics desperately want to maintain. Their comments reflect a new emerging discourse of nurses in academia and reveal their interpersonal experiences of working in an academic setting.

In chapter 7, four nursing faculty from The University of Louisiana at Lafayette describe their experiences during fall semester 2005 after Hurricane Katrina hit the Gulf Coast. Gwen Leigh explains how faculty managed their personal challenges. Jill Laroussini tells how she balanced resourcefulness and flexibility while maintaining academic commitments. Sudha C. Patel and Ardith L. Sudduth describe their strategies for helping students cope. The authors share how they responded to a state of crisis while maintaining their educational commitments to students.

Ruth Neese, Gene Majka, and Geneiva Tennant, in chapter 8, explore the implications of three global challenges: (1) the brain drain of educated professionals migrating from less to more developed countries, (2) the shortage of nursing faculty, and (3) the relationship of literacy and nursing students. The authors describe the global nature of these challenges for nursing education, explain how American educators are affected by them, and offer local strategies teachers can use to meet these global challenges. Beyond raising the consciousness of U.S. nurse educators about how these global situations impinge on their professional lives, the chapter offers suggestions for action at the local, national, and international levels.

Benchmarking involves identifying processes or practices from other institutions and then using them to help an organization improve similar processes or practices. Benchmarking answers questions such as: "How are we doing in comparison with other schools" and "Who is using the best practices and what can we learn from them?" Diane M. Billings, in chapter 9, reviews four types of benchmarking practices, steps that are common to most benchmarking activities, and how to integrate benchmarking into education practices in a school of nursing. This is a good chapter to read to learn about benchmarking and its use in nursing education programs.

In Part III of the ARNE, chapters shift to initiatives that enhance learning and student development; some of these rely on new technology and others focus on guided assessment. We begin Part III with a chapter by Ramona Nelson on student support services essential in a distance education program. Distance education has become an increasingly effective tool in meeting the educational needs of students seeking degrees in nursing. A quality, online education program requires a well-designed curriculum as well as a wide range of student support services. Examples of key student support services include academic advising, bookstore services, financial aid, and library services. This chapter describes required online student support services, explains how these online services can be structured, and identifies resources for developing them.

In chapter 11, Linda Felver and Catherine Van Son describe the educational innovations they developed as part of their Older Adult Focus Project, intended to increase the ability of nurses to provide care for older adults. As part of that project, they created materials to build into an existing online baccalaureate program for registered nurses. They also developed a stand-alone CD-ROM to assist nursing students and nurses to increase their abilities in working with older adults and to assist educators who want to infuse older adult content into existing courses or teach it as a separate course. They describe the development process they used, which can be adapted to other educational settings.

Chapter 12 describes how to use a course management system (CMS) to enrich student learning and enhance teaching. A CMS is a web-based "frame" through which faculty can communicate with students; distribute information; and facilitate the exchange of ideas, information, and resources. Linda M. Goodfellow explains how to use a CMS to manage courses taught in a school of nursing, describes innovative ways of using a CMS in both a traditional and virtual classroom, and examines the significant role of a CMS in nursing education.

In chapter 13, Janice M. Jones, Kay Sackett, W. Scott Erdley, and John B. Blyth describe how to develop electronic portfolios (or ePortfolios). By preparing an ePortfolio, students can communicate their accomplishments and competencies, have an opportunity to work with technology, and demonstrate their ability to use information technology as a tool. The authors describe their project to prepare nursing students for professional practice by using a technology-based format showcasing students' talents and skills in the form of ePortfolios. In addition, the advantages and disadvantages of implementing ePortfolios are discussed, and the authors share many of their tools with readers.

In chapter 14, Paulette Demaske Rollant reviews the literature on predictors and tools to identify students at risk for failure on the NCLEX-RN®. In this chapter, she presents interventions she has used over the years to successfully prepare students for the licensure examination and for taking other tests in nursing programs. These simple interventions can be used by faculty to prepare students to be successful test takers in nursing programs.

The goal of the ARNE is to keep you updated on innovations and new ideas in nursing education. We hope you agree that volume 5 met that goal. We appreciate the hard work of the authors who, as teacher-scholars, so generously share their innovations for the benefit of educators everywhere. A heartfelt thanks to you for reading and recommending the *Annual Review of Nursing Education* to other nurse educators!

Marilyn H. Oermann, Editor
Kathleen T. Heinrich, Associate Editor

REFERENCE

Hu, W. (2006, April 16). "New York leads politeness trend? Get outta here." *The New York Times*, p. 1.

Part I

Clinical Nursing Education: New Directions in Assessment and Clinical Experiences for Students

Chapter 1

Standardized Patients in Nursing Education

Louise Sherman Jenkins and Kathy Schaivone

Educators in nursing face multiple challenges in planning effective learning experiences and providing constructive, objective evaluation of knowledge and skills in learners. Competition for clinical sites, increasing complexity and acuity levels of patients in clinical settings, and heightened levels of public concern about patient safety are key among factors that mandate learners in health professions demonstrate clinical competence prior to entering the actual clinical setting. Integration of standardized patients (SPs) into learning experiences can help educators overcome some of these barriers to effective clinical teaching and evaluation. This sophisticated form of simulation allows learners to practice skills with a real person in a safe and controlled environment. Having these simulated patients highly trained to portray focused scenarios allows for consistency of experiences across learners and strengthens the reliability of the evaluation process. Consistency of clinical experience and evaluation of learners is maintained through the use of trained SPs portraying scenarios tailored specifically to the objectives of the encounter.

At the University of Maryland School of Nursing, high value is placed on the integration of simulation into nursing curricula, beginning in the classroom, extending through laboratory experiences with various types of simulation incorporating various types of models ranging from simple to exceedingly complex (Morton & Rauen, 2004).

This chapter was accepted on April 6, 2006.

During the late 1990s, the University of Maryland Schools of Nursing and Medicine were using SPs on a limited basis with students. At that time, the SPs were contracted from another university with an established program. A thorough needs assessment conducted by both schools indicated that the education and evaluation of students could be expanded and enhanced if the campus had its own SP program. Both schools agreed a strong collaborative relationship in this endeavor would have rich mutual benefits for the learners, the two schools, and the University of Maryland academic health science campus. In late 2000, the SP program began operation as the Clinical Education and Evaluation Laboratory, a joint venture of the Schools of Nursing and Medicine.

This chapter contains a definition of SPs, a general discussion of integrating SP encounters into nursing curricula, and background information of the origins and evolution of the SP's role in medical and nursing education. Turning attention to the SP laboratory, the physical environment is described as well as the operation of the facility. In the section about SP encounters, we describe various models for SP encounters, explicate the role of the educator, discuss case writing and evaluation of learners, training of SPs, and the process of the actual SP encounter. Learner performance and the role of the SP, the learner, and the educator are described. Also included is a discussion of how learners and educators evaluate the SP encounter, and how SPs are evaluated, as well as how the SP program is evaluated. Finally, implications for educators using SPs in nursing are discussed. Throughout the chapter, we offer general information about using SPs and our experiences in the Clinical Education and Evaluation Laboratory to discuss the approaches used in these various areas.

Background

What Is a Standardized Patient?

The Association of Standardized Patient Educators defines a SP as "a person trained to portray a patient: This can be for instruction, assessment, or practice of communication and/or examining skills of a health care provider" (Gliva-McConvey, 2006). Training of SPs is key and should result in:

...a person who has been carefully coached to simulate an actual patient so accurately that the simulation cannot be detected by a skilled clinician. In performing the simulation, the SP presents the gestalt of the patient being simulated; not just the history, but the body language, the physical findings, and the emotional and personality characteristics as well (Barrows, 1987).

Standardized patients are lay people/actors who are employed by a center or laboratory, carefully trained to simulate a particular "case" or script, and—in many cases—provide feedback to the learner on their performance.

Integrating Standardized Patient Encounters Into Nursing Curricula

Standardized Patient encounters can be integrated into the curriculum for instruction and practice of skills, to evaluate learners, for program evaluation, faculty development, and research. Standardized Patient encounters allow for repeated experiences in which the learner can attend to the critical aspects of the situation and improve performance in response to patient outcomes, feedback, or both. There are characteristics of SP encounters that lend themselves to effective integration into nursing education.

The learner is an active participant in the experience rather than a passive observer. Because these encounters take place in the safe and predictable environment of a laboratory, errors are educational experiences rather than patient disasters. In a clinical setting, the experiences of learners are often uneven and controlled by the availability and condition of patients. In SP encounters, the behavior, presentation, and responses by the patient are determined by the case, and the patients are trained to adhere to that training. The sessions are flexible in that they can take place at the convenience of the educator and learners. Through this methodology, educators can do direct comparisons of learner competence and efficiently use their time by observing multiple learners in one setting. The SP evaluations are responsive to real differences in performance due to case control. Learners can receive immediate feedback and debriefing from SPs and educators.

During SP sessions in which the learner is challenged with advanced clinical management of complex patient problems, educators are able to view the continuum of a student's ability to take a history, complete an appropriate physical examination, plan for appropriate interventions, and use some basic care measures with the SP. Through the integration of SP encounters in the curriculum, universal competencies that are the foundation of skills needed for effective clinician—patient interactions can be taught and assessed. Ideally, a decision to integrate SP encounters into a course or program would occur during development of the course. Doing so allows for careful identification of cognitive, psychomotor, and affective knowledge and skills to be specified in the learning objectives. Integrating an SP encounter(s) into the curriculum serves as a focal point for the development and integration of competency-based skill evaluation. Standardized Patient encounters can also be added into existing courses and programs as an innovative teaching strategy as well as an assessment strategy. In addition, the SP encounter offers an opportunity to use knowledge and skills attained in an appropriate context.

Origin and Evolution of the Role

Over 40 years ago, Dr. Howard Barrows—a neurologist wanting to better assess the clinical skills of his students—became the "father" of simulated patients as he employed and trained actors who were readily available in southern California to work with his students. Using cases of actual neurology patients as templates for the scenarios the actors would portray, a detailed script was developed to determine the exact detail of each case to be presented. Thus, these simulated "patients" were trained to present the same signs, symptoms, history, emotional state, and, in some cases, physical examination findings to students.

This approach allowed Dr. Barrows to present the same "patient" multiple times for his students. He could then observe each student with the simulated patient in a safe and controlled environment and assess the competency of each student under the exact same set of circumstances. These simulated patients were trained to provide feedback to students on their performance. Simulated patients became known as "standardized" patients, a term coined by Canadian psychometrician Geoffrey Norman, and this umbrella term for the numerous variations of the SP role serves to the present (Wallace, 2006).

Standardized Patients in Medical Education

Standardized Patients are widely used in medical education, with nearly every medical school in the country having its own facility. Literature in medicine is replete with numerous reports of the uses and effectiveness of working with SPs in medical education. A number of studies examining the effectiveness of SP encounters have demonstrated that use of SPs provides high-fidelity simulation of real clinical situations (Colliver & Swartz, 1997). A consensus statement presented at the Association of American Medical Colleges Consensus Conference on the Use of Standardized Patients in the Teaching and Evaluation of Clinical Skills asserted, "...fifteen years of research on the evaluation of clinical competence support the recommendation to use multiple SPs as an adjunct to current evaluation method" (Anderson & Kassebaum, 1993, p. 475). The study documented that SPs, when used in conjunction with other educational evaluation data, can substantially improve the quality of information for formative and summative evaluation of students.

As this body of evidence has expanded, and licensing boards acknowledged a growing demand by consumers, hospitals, and residency programs to ensure the clinical competency of students graduating from medical school, the National Board of Medical Examiners (NBME) conducted research on the feasibility of using SPs in the licensure process. Following years of research and testing, the NBME determined SP encounters to be valid and reliable in the assessment of student competence.

In July 2004, the U.S. Medical Licensing Examination was expanded to include not only a written test of clinical knowledge but also a step 2 Clinical Skills examination (CSE). The CSE is a multistation examination during which the candidate participates in 12 SP encounters. The CSE is scored in three sections: (1) integrated clinical encounter, (2) communication and interpersonal skills, and (3) spoken English proficiency. Passing all three sections of the CSE is required to become licensed to practice medicine in the United States (Federation of State Medical Boards of the United States and NBME, 2005). Although there are detractors and concerns raised by the American Medical Association and the American Medical Student Association, the CSE examination is providing a mechanism to evaluate student skills and ultimately to improve medical education and physician quality.

Standardized Patients in Nursing Education

Although there seems to be growing interest and implementation of the use of SPs in nursing education, progress has been slow. Results of an informal Internet survey of SP facilities conducted by the authors in 2003 revealed that only 17 of those were working with nursing students at any level; 15 of the 17 SP facilities were in the United States. There are few publications about SPs found in the nursing literature to date. One of the earliest of these was a report in which nursing students viewed a video produced with faculty demonstrating physical assessment skills with "simulated" patients (Lincoln, Layton, & Holdman, 1978) before they practiced these skills on each other. In this case, the simulated patients were used as a teaching strategy. Yoo and Yoo (2003) reported on using SPs for teaching several fundamental nursing skills, as well as communication with undergraduate students.

Examples of SPs working with graduate students include reports with psychosocial nurse practitioner students (O'Connor, Albert, & Thomas, 1999); adult and pediatric nurse practitioners (Vessey & Huss, 2002); adult nurse practitioners receiving instruction via video teleconferencing (Seibert, Guthrie, & Adamo, 2004); family nurse practitioners (Ebbert & Conners, 2004); and nurse practitioner students being assessed for cultural competency (Rutledge, Garzon, Scott, & Karlowicz, 2004). Only one report (Konkle-Parker, Cramer, & Hamill, 2002) was found describing the use of SPs with learners in an in-service setting.

Standardized Patient Laboratory

Physical Environment

Standardized patient encounters typically take place in a laboratory. This setting offers a realistic setting for simulating clinical care situations as well as a safe environment for learning, practicing, and evaluating learners. The laboratory setting also allows for standardized, reproducible, consistent encounters across learners. These facilities are typically constructed with multiple examination rooms equipped with digital video cameras and microphones for recording. Historically, these centers were located in and operated by schools of medicine. Increasingly, a number of existing and new centers are now interdisciplinary and may also house other simulation activities.

At the University of Maryland, the SP laboratory, the Clinical Education and Evaluation Laboratory (CEEL), is a joint venture of the University of Maryland Schools of Medicine and Nursing. The CEEL is a state-of-the-art facility dedicated to the teaching, assessment, and evaluation of clinical skills. The mission of the laboratory is to provide an innovative setting for learners to enhance clinical skills or participate in a formative or summative evaluation process. Priority learners are nursing and medical students, although as noted later in this chapter, other types of learners are served. The CEEL is housed in the School of Nursing and has six examination rooms equipped with video and audio recording. Outside each examination room is a charting station equipped with Internet access for students to use with their laptop computers for charting or completing postencounter evaluations.

The CEEL facility includes an office for staff, an observation/training room with television monitors, and a small SP break area. Access to classrooms located in the same wing allows for orientation of learners and training of SPs. Additionally, a physiologically competent computerized human patient simulator in the CEEL provides options for blended simulation of invasive techniques that can be integrated into the SP encounter. The CEEL is used for teaching, skill acquisition, clinical competency assessment, and research; thus, it serves as a critical resource for the academic health science campus.

Operation of the SP Laboratory

The CEEL is directed collaboratively by an educator from the School of Nursing and one from the School of Medicine. Two full-time employees, a managing director and a coordinator, staff the CEEL. A full roster of more than 80 SPs is employed and available to work according to scheduled needs for training and SP encounters. The SPs are diverse in many ways including gender, ethnic background, language spoken, physical characteristics, and age, which ranges from 4 to 80 years. The staff hires, trains, evaluates, and schedules SPs. They collaborate with educators in case development, implementation, and support of learner evaluations. Additionally, they work with educators to orient, schedule, and evaluate learners for their SP encounters and provide data collection services.

Although housed in the School of Nursing, costs of construction of the CEEL, all equipment, salaries, and operating expenses are shared equally between the Schools of Nursing and Medicine. Each school is billed separately for costs of SP training and encounters with their respective students. Student costs are included in their tuition. Other programs and schools on the campus may use the CEEL as scheduling allows; however, they are billed at a higher rate, as are external users of the facility.

Standardized Patient Encounters

Models of Standardized Patient Encounters

The most common model for SP encounters is a 1:1 interaction between learner and SP. Because this encounter lends itself to experiences that are designed for skill acquisition and/or evaluation of learner performance and competence, evaluation of the experience can be either formative or summative. Over time, a new model that allowed learners to move from one SP to another in a series of scenarios was termed an Objective Structured Clinical Examination in which the learner moves from SP station to SP station to perform specific skills in a focused encounter. This model is widely used today in medical schools and, to a much lesser extent, in nursing education. Objective Structured Clinical Examination encounters are more typically used for summative evaluation and competency testing.

At the CEEL, the traditional SP encounter is widely used by educators in nursing. This model is frequently expanded to include a parent/child dyad for learners in pediatrics and family practice. Another modification of this model is multiple learners and one SP in an encounter. An example of the use of this model is a unique program focused on interprofessional, patient care planning that involved learners from nursing, medicine, pharmacy, and dentistry. In addition, blended simulation, a model used at the CEEL since 2001, is increasingly being used. Blended encounters allow the learner to move from SP to human patient simulator in the same encounter so that both invasive and noninvasive skills and competencies can be incorporated into the encounter.

A final model of SP encounter currently in use by the CEEL takes the SP into the classroom setting. In this experience, the educator models desired behavior(s) (e.g., interviewing a psychiatric patient) with an SP. Learners can observe, then rotate participation with the SP while the educator assumes a coaching role. A useful process in this model is the ability to call "time out" at intervals; this allows other learners in the encounter to probe the interviewer's thoughts, ideas, and strategies while the SP "freezes" or "suspends" until "time in" is called.

As can be seen, SPs work with learners in a variety of capacities, such as formative exercises for interviewing, physical examination assessment, and challenging communication scenarios. Examples of various types of SP encounters regularly offered by the CEEL for learners in undergraduate and graduate nursing programs are found in Table 1.1.Variations on the SP models presented allow for use of SPs with learners in a variety of other courses, continuing education and faculty development efforts, as well as in research by doctoral students and educators.

Educator Role

Educators participate in every aspect of SP encounters. They are responsible for case writing, development of assessment tools, checking the quality of SP training and performance, and participating in evaluation of students. A key to successful SP encounters is a direct result of the goals and objectives established by the educator prior to the development of the session and their collaboration in assessment of student performance.

Cases that are used in SP encounters are carefully planned with input from the educator(s) for a particular course or program. This process begins several months in advance to allow for planning, training, and scheduling. At the CEEL, the educator completes the SP Encounter Request Form that covers the multiple small details that need to be determined to tailor the case specifically to the desired objectives for the encounter. This form is reviewed, and appropriate approvals for required resources are obtained.

Case Writing

The development of an effective SP case requires significant time and planning prior to the implementation of a project. The task of the learner and the goals and objectives of the session must be clearly defined. Educators should determine if the SP encounter will be most effective as practice or assessment of learner skills. The specific behaviors the

TABLE 1.1   Examples of Regular SP Encounters at the Clinical Education and Evaluation Laboratory

Examples from Courses	Type of Encounter	Target Skills/Behaviors	Type of Evaluation	SP Model
Undergraduate-Level Courses				
Communication module	Interview and therapeutic communication	Interview/history taking; Communication and interpersonal skills	Summative	1 Learner—1 SP
Maternal child health	Interview and postpartum physical examination	Interview/history taking; Communication and interpersonal skills; Problem solving; Counseling	Formative	1 Learner—1 SP
Senior practicum in women's health	Interview and post partum examination	Interview/history taking; Communication and interpersonal skills; Problem solving; Counseling	Summative	1 Learner—1 SP
Mental health	Interview and counseling	Interview/history taking; Communication and interpersonal skills; Problem solving; Counseling	Formative	1 SP in classroom
Graduate-Level Courses				
Physical assessment	Head-to-toe examination	Interview/history taking; Communication and interpersonal skills; Physical examination skills	Formative	1 Learner—1 SP

TABLE 1.1 (*continued*)

Adult NP Family NP	Focused H&P	Interview/history taking; Communication and interpersonal skills; Physical examination skills; Diagnosis; Management	Summative	1 Learner—1 SP
Pediatrics and FNP physical assessment	Well child examination	Interview/history taking; Communication and interpersonal skills; Physical examination skills	Formative	1 Learner— Mother/child SPs
Mental health	Interview and counseling	Interview/history taking; Communication and interpersonal skills; Counseling	Formative	1 Learner—1 SP
Mental health	Interview and counseling	Interview/history taking; Communication and interpersonal skills; Problem solving; Counseling; Diagnosis; Management	Summative	1 Learner—SP family members
Adult NP Family NP	Blended simulation focused H&P with SP and physical examination skills of human patient simulator	Interview/history taking; Communication and interpersonal skills; Physical examination skills; Problem solving; Diagnosis; Management	Summative	1 Learner—1 SP

FNP, family nurse practitioner; H&P, history & physical; NP, nurse practitioner; SP, standardized patient.

learner needs to demonstrate should also be built into the case—clinical skills, communication skills, or both. Finally, a plan is developed for postencounter, such as writing up notes of the session.

The construction of an SP case includes a synopsis, opening statement, signs and symptoms to be exhibited, history, affect, and patient behavior. The role of the SP in the encounter is defined in the case and in subsequent training sessions, along with specific details regarding information that can be given to the learner. In addition, working from the perspective of the "patient" they are portraying, the SP gives constructive feedback to the learners that may include aspects of both verbal and nonverbal communication, as well as the target knowledge and skills such as performing a physical examination. During case development, articulation of the behaviors or skills the learner is to practice or demonstrate are defined along with the assessment of interpersonal skills. The educator reviews and approves the written case, "pilot tests" the case with SPs, and finally approves or participates in revising as needed.

Training of Standardized Patients

Success or failure of an encounter is determined to a large extent upon the training of the SP(s). Standardized patients need careful and consistent training to ensure their reliability and accuracy of the portrayal of the case and their assessment of students. SPs are provided with a case/scenario to memorize prior to training for an encounter. Several hours of training and rehearsal with the SPs are required prior to working with students. Training should be done by expert SP trainers; in the CEEL, this is the managing director who has extensive experience in this area. This training may be done individually or with a small group of SPs—this is sometimes referred to as an SP "team" for a particular case—those who may be portraying the cases concurrently.

Attention is given to: (1) specific verbal and nonverbal behaviors appropriate for the role, (2) a detailed review of case information, and (3) directives regarding how to answer learner questions and what information can or cannot be provided. Video recordings of prior encounters, as well as observation of others performing the role in an examination, may be used in training as well as informal role-playing. After training for the case and the evaluation form to be used, both the case and the form are piloted with the educator(s). Feedback from this piloting helps ensure that both the content and the portrayal of the patient are realistic. This training process helps ensure consistent and realistic portrayal of the patient role and reliable and accurate completion of an assessment checklist.

Encounter and Preparation of Students

Educators begin to prepare learners for their SP encounters by sharing the objective(s) for the session, expectations for appropriate dress and equipment (e.g., stethoscope), and scheduled date and time for the encounter. Learners are reminded that, although SPs are feigning a condition, disease, or problem, they are not feigning being a human being; thus, they are to be treated as an actual patient. At the scheduled time of the encounter, learners come to the CEEL where they participate in an orientation session lasting about 10 minutes. At this time, they complete video consent forms, video labels, and receive their room/patient assignments. Information is given about time, warning bells, where to complete the self-assessment, evaluation, relevant documentation, feedback session procedures, as well as a description of their case.

Learners move into the hall outside their assigned room/patient and read the patient case record. They are instructed when to enter the room and proceed with the assigned case. After the SP encounter, learners complete the self-assessment forms, then re-enter their encounter room where the SP provides feedback on the learner's performance. Any other documentation, such as charting, is completed following feedback. In most cases, the learner returns all materials to CEEL staff and leaves with the video of their encounter. They are asked to return these videos after they have been viewed.

Evaluation of Learners

A major benefit of an SP encounter is the ability to have the learner's performance, whether for formative or summative evaluation of knowledge and skills, carefully reviewed from multiple perspectives. Depending on the goal and objective of each case, evaluation materials, including competency assessments, need to be developed and tested prior to the case with careful attention to pilot-testing, training of those who will use the materials in the evaluation process, and estimation of reliability and validity as appropriate (Oermann & Gaberson, 2006, p. 244). The sources of evaluation include the SP, the educator, and self-evaluation by the learner. First, the SP provides immediate feedback in the form of a verbal debriefing, and this is offered from the perspective of the patient. SP training for each case includes focusing on how to provide constructive feedback to learners. SPs are also carefully trained to evaluate the particular competencies developed for the case. Just as consistency of cases is a key component of SP encounters across students, consistency of SP ratings is assessed on a regular basis. This is done both informally by CEEL staff and formally at regular intervals.

Educators are strongly encouraged to be in the observation area of the CEEL facility where they can monitor performance of up to six students concurrently. In addition, educators have the opportunity to review the video of each SP encounter. Learners can review their video-tape either individually or with an educator. This self-evaluation serves as a powerful reinforcement of the evaluations provided by the SP and educator.

Standardized patient encounters provide a unique opportunity for students to receive immediate feedback from the patient they have just seen. Clinical feedback is described by Ende (1983) as "information describing students' performance in a given activity that is intended to guide their future performance in that same or related activity. It is a key step in the acquisition of clinical skills" (p. 777). To enable SPs to participate in the learner's acquisition of skills, they are trained to provide verbal and written feedback to students. The written feedback is usually in a checklist format. The content of the checklist is determined during the project planning and development. It can include assessment of history taking, communication, and interpersonal and counseling skills. With precise training, SPs can accurately assess a broad range of skills.

Development of the SP feedback tool is based on the objectives set for overall learner assessment during case construction. Typically SPs assess the learner's ability to establish and maintain rapport, interact in a professional manner, and use appropriate questioning and information-sharing skills. Questions such as, "Did the student make you feel comfortable and respected during the encounter?" help the SP speak from the perspective of the character they have been portraying and determine how that character felt about the learner during their time together.

Standardized patients complete a written checklist and then give one-to-one feedback to the learner immediately following the encounter. The manner in which the verbal feedback is given is also standardized. SPs follow a format beginning with, "This is the opportunity when I get to tell you what it was like to be your patient and have you as my health care provider." By immediately asking questions such as "How do you think it went?" followed by saying "Tell me two things you thought you did well and two things you want to improve next time," the SP facilitates discussion. Their feedback is always given in a constructive and thoughtful manner, as SPs are trained to express how they felt using "I" messages the learner can readily understand. Examples of these statements are: "I felt neglected when you answered two phone calls during my time with you" or "I felt respected when you carefully draped me so that I was not unnecessarily exposed during the physical exam." This feedback is nonjudgmental and based on learner behavior, because the learner needs to understand how they are perceived by their patient.

It is important to provide the tools for the SPs to identify objectively the behaviors demonstrated by learners. Although SP feedback may have an element of subjectivity, the key is to stress to the learners that this evaluation can be helpful to their development of competence in the skills addressed in the encounter.

Standardized patients are providing clinical skills feedback to students with increasing frequency. For example, at the CEEL, SPs assess the accuracy of a student pulmonary examination during a focused asthma encounter. Skills such as auscultation and testing of tactile fremitis can be accurately assessed by the SPs once they are trained in correct and incorrect procedures and given the opportunity to practice the encounter with faculty members. Such feedback offers a valuable resource to faculty and enhances the overall evaluation process.

Evaluation by Learners

All learners participating in SP encounters are asked to evaluate the experience. A 5-point scale (1 = strongly disagree to 5 = strongly agree) was used to rate extent of agreement with eight statements about the encounter as seen in Figure 1.1. Over the years of the CEEL's operation, which currently conducts more than 3,200 SP encounters per year, these ratings have been consistently very positive with mean ratings ranging

CLINICAL EDUCATION AND EVALUATION LABORATORY
University of Maryland Baltimore

Date of your encounter_____

Using the code below, please circle the number that indicates the extent to which you agree with each of the following statements:

5 = Strongly Agree   1 = Strongly Disagree

1) I feel the encounter with the standardized patient(s) was realistic.
       5   4   3   2   1

2) I feel the encounter with the standardized patient(s) was a good measure of my knowledge.
       5   4   3   2   1

3) I feel the encounter with the standardized patient(s) was a good measure of my skills.
       5   4   3   2   1

4) I feel the encounter with the standardized patient(s) was a useful learning experience.

       5   4   3   2   1

5) I feel the feedback provided by the standardized patient(s) was constructive.
       5   4   3   2   1

6) I feel the encounter with the standardized patient(s) strengthened my confidence in my own abilities.
       5   4   3   2   1

7) I feel the encounter with the standardized patient(s) improved my comfort in performing the activities involved.
       5   4   3   2   1

8) I feel the encounter with the standardized patient(s) was valuable.
       5   4   3   2   1

••

My overall impression of the Clinical Education and Evaluation Lab is:

Comments:

FIGURE 1.1   Learner evaluation of standardized patient encounter.
Source: Clinical Education and Evaluation Laboratory, University of Maryland Baltimore, 2001, revised 2003. Reprinted by permission, April 10, 2006.

from 4.43–4.55; estimates of Cronbach's alpha range from 0.89 to 0.93. There is also room on the form for learners to write in their overall impressions of the laboratory, as well as to add comments.

Although these comments are consistently overwhelmingly positive, there was also some indication of learner anxiety prior to the SP encounter. This feedback prompted development and implementation of a computer-based orientation module. Some educators use this module in the classroom to prepare their students whereas others make their learners aware of this resource available for individual review.

Evaluation by Educators

Evaluation of SP encounters by educators is consistently sought. Although informal approaches were used in the early days of the CEEL, now all educators who work with the CEEL in developing and implementing SP encounters for their learners are asked to complete an online survey to provide feedback on their experience. A series of questions addresses the value of various aspects of the encounter, including the video, as well as educator satisfaction with things such as SP training, quality of SP feedback, SP evaluation of learners, and aspects of the CEEL operation. Space is allowed for comments and constructive suggestions as well. To date, these responses have been overwhelmingly positive; the lowest level of satisfaction is in flexibility of scheduling SP encounters for learners. In all cases, first priority is given to nursing and medical learners; however, with large numbers of learners in each of these schools, there sometimes needs to be some negotiation to accommodate needs for scheduling.

Evaluation of Standardized Patients

Training does not end once the SP enters the examination room or classroom. Ongoing evaluation of SP performance ensures continuous quality improvement and is reinforced by ongoing training for the SP. A structured performance appraisal should be conducted frequently on all SPs. Each assessment should be based on the goals and objectives of the performance of the SP and typically includes accuracy of information given, consistency of the SP across all the learners they work with for a particular project, careful delivery of content and refraining from volunteering information, physical portrayal, ability to stay in character, and accuracy and reliability of SP completed checklists. As in learner assessment, SP assessment should be as objective as possible.

In high-stakes projects, SP programs may choose to assess inter-rater reliability to estimate accuracy of checklist completion. This requires multiple SPs trained on a case and rotation of the role of these individuals as observer and patient. Having one SP observe and rate performance of another can be an effective method of continuous quality control. The completion of two evaluation forms for each learner allows for calculation of percentage of agreement between the SPs. In the CEEL, the target is 95%–100% agreement across SPs evaluating learners in a given scenario. Review of taped encounters can also be used in this process.

Program Evaluation

Continuous performance improvement and the creative use of technology are the cornerstones of the laboratory. Drawing on principles used by numerous businesses (Pande, Neuman, & Cavanaugh, 2000), key points included in the ongoing evaluation of the SP program at the University of Maryland follow:

- Ensuring linkage of SP encounter to institutional and educational objectives;
- Prioritizing of the demonstrated need for SP encounters relative to other initiatives, programs, and priorities;
- Using facts and data to address student and institutional performance and to support actions at all levels of decision-making;
- Creating accountabilities, expectations, roles, and responsibilities for the organization;
- Conducting regular reviews of student performance; and
- Ensuring visible, active feedback mechanisms to learners, educators, and programs.

Implications for Educators

Throughout this discussion, numerous advantages of working with SPs as teaching and assessment strategies—including convenience, flexibility in scheduling, specificity to precise objectives, and being reproducible across learners—are evident. Cases can be tailored to the class, program, curriculum, or testing situation, and are consistent for all learners. SPs, unlike actual patients, can be available anytime and, although typically in a laboratory facility such as the CEEL, be any place, such as a classroom. Learners become actively involved in the encounter whether it is for skill acquisition or competency evaluation. Those learners needing remediation can be identified early on so that strategies can be planned to help them prepare for working with real patients in the clinical setting. Because efforts are made to ensure the reliability and validity of assessment data, the information from SP encounters yields high value for the learner, as well as for other facets of teaching and learning (Epstein & Hundert, 2002).

The major limitations of working with SPs are the time needed for careful planning, training, and scheduling, and evaluation of actual encounters, as well as the resources needed to support a facility for SP activity and the operation of the program. These factors are likely the major reasons why educators in nursing have not been rapid adopters of working with SPs. Although it may be tempting to resort to role-play as a substitute strategy, the precision of the experience ensured by the careful planning, the exacting scenario to which the SP is trained, the multiple sources of evaluation information, and the video capability of a laboratory setting are lost in the process. Likewise, having learners practice various skills on each other can compromise modesty, privacy, and, in the worst-case scenario, pose considerable liability.

Educators not having an SP facility in their setting do have several options available to them. First, check if there is a facility nearby and contact that facility to explore options for a possible working relationship. Many facilities will work with educators to provide the needed SP encounters for a fee. This approach could be especially needed to educators in the clinical setting who desire to have newly employed nurses tested for competency in relevant areas or to evaluate the outcomes of classes or workshops. Nearly every medical school now has its own SP facility, and many of these operate as an interprofessional laboratory. If they do not have capacity in their setting, educators might explore working with existing facilities in developing cases and hiring SPs from their program to come to their setting for SP encounters. This would require the ability to simulate the desired setting although the video capability may not be available; not having this would compromise the ability of learners to self-evaluate from the video of the encounter.

Summary

This chapter focused on the highest level of fidelity or consistency with real situations for which learners are being prepared on the simulation continuum. Working with SPs to provide learners with experiences that can optimize learning, be as consistent and objective as possible and facilitate the transition of knowledge and skills, which allow for a more competent and confident clinician to enter the clinical arena for safe care of real patients in a clinical setting.

That said, the continuing nursing shortage and escalating faculty shortage have placed heavy demands on educators in nursing who seek to maintain the highest quality education possible for their learners. Multiple pressures and demands on faculty time for teaching, advisement, clinical work, research, and community service increasingly mean that creativity will be key to maintaining quality nursing education programs. Resourceful educators will need to utilize multiple teaching strategies and select those that allow students to demonstrate a range of skills. The integration of valid methodologies will allow schools of nursing to prepare competent, professional, caring, and creative nurses. Whereas integration of SPs into the curriculum and other types of learning experiences is not a substitute for learning experiences in clinical settings, we believe it can make a significant contribution toward this goal with learners in academic as well as other professional settings.

REFERENCES

Anderson, J. A., & Kassebaum, D. G. (1993). Proceedings of the AAMC's consensus conference on the use of standardized patients in the teaching and evaluation of clinical skills. *Academic Medicine, 68*(6), 437–478.

Barrows, H. S. (1987). *Association of Standardized Patient Educators.* Retrieved January 10, 2006, from http://www.aspeducators.org/sp_info.htm

Colliver, J. A., & Swartz, M. H. (1997). Assessing clinical performance with standardized patients. *Journal of the American Medical Association, 278,* 790–791.

Ebbert, D. W., & Conners, H. (2004). Standardized patient experiences: Evaluation of clinical performance and nurse practitioner student satisfaction. *Nursing Education Perspectives, 25*(1), 2–5.

Ende, J. (1983). Feedback in clinical medical education. *Journal of the American Medical Association, 250,* 777–781.

Epstein, R. M., & Hundert, E. M. (2002). Defining and assessing professional competence. *Journal of the American Medical Association, 287*, 225–235.

Federation of State Medical Boards of the United States, Inc., and National Board of Medical Examiners. (2005). United States Medical Licensure Examination. Retrieved March 28, 2006, from http://www.usmle.org/step2/Step2CS/Step2CS2006GI/TOC.asp

Gliva-McConvey, G. (2006). What is a standardized patient? *Association of Standardized Patient Educators.* Retrieved January 10, 2006, from http://www.aspeducators.org/sp_info.htm

Konkle-Parker, D. J., Cramer, C. K., & Hamill, C. (2002). Standardized patient training: A modality for teaching interviewing skills. *The Journal of Continuing Education in Nursing, 33*, 225–230.

Lincoln, R., Layton, J., & Holdman, H. (1978). Using simulated patients to teach assessment. *Nursing Outlook, 26*, 316–320.

Morton, P. G., & Rauen, C. A. (2004). Using simulation in nursing education: The University of Maryland and Georgetown University experiences. In M.H. Oermann & K.T. Heinrich (Eds.), *Annual Review of Nursing Education* (Vol. 2, pp. 139–161). New York: Springer Publishing.

O'Connor, F. W., Albert, M. L., & Thomas, M. D. (1999). Incorporating standardized patients into a psychosocial nurse practitioner program. *Archives of Psychiatric Nursing, 13*, 240–247.

Oermann, M. H., & Gaberson, K. B. (2006). *Evaluation and testing in nursing education* (2nd ed.). New York: Springer Publishing.

Pande, P. S., Neuman, R. P., & Cavanaugh, R. R. (2000). *The six-sigma way: How GE, Motorola, and other top companies are honing their performance.* New York: McGraw-Hill.

Rutledge, C. M., Garzon, L., Scott, M., & Karlowicz, K. (2004). Using standardized patients to teach and evaluate nurse practitioner students on cultural competency. *International Journal of Nursing Education Scholarship, 1*(1). Retrieved January 10, 2006, from http://www.bepress.com/cgi/viewcontent.cgi?article=1048&context=ijnes

Seibert, D. C., Guthrie, J. T., & Adamo, G. (2004). Improving learning outcomes: Integration of standardized patients and telemedicine technology. *Nursing Education Perspectives, 25*, 232–237.

Vessey, J. A., & Huss, K . (2002). Using standardized patients in advanced practice nursing education. *Journal of Professional Nursing, 18*(1), 29–35.

Wallace, P. (2006). Following the threads of an innovation: The history of standardized patients in medical education. Retrieved January 10, 2006, from http://www.aspeducators.org/sp_info.htm

Yoo, M. S., & Yoo, I. Y. (2003). The effectiveness of standardized patients as a teaching method for nursing fundamentals. *Journal of Nursing Education, 42*, 444–448.

Chapter 2

A Multidimensional Strategy for Teaching Cultural Competence: Spotlight on an Innovative Field Trip Experience

Marianne R. Jeffreys, Lenore Bertone, Jo-Ann Douglas, Vivien Li, and Sara Newman

Providing culturally specific, quality nursing care for increasingly diverse populations is a growing professional challenge. The expanding number of minority and immigrant populations seeking health care compounded by the growing diverse nursing student population predicted in the future suggest that increasingly nurses will care for patients who are "culturally different." Culturally different patients are patients whose racial, ethnic, gender, socioeconomic, and/or religious backgrounds and/or identities are different from the student or nurse. For educators, preparing culturally diverse nursing students and nurses to care competently for culturally different patients will be even more complex. One added challenge is to provide innovative, meaningful educational opportunities to enhance the cultural competency of health care professionals so that they can positively transform health care. Advanced practice nurses are in a key position to create positive changes (Jeffreys, 2002, 2005, 2006).

Nurse educators are expected to prepare advanced practice nurses who are equipped to actively transform health care practice, education, research, and policy to meet the needs of culturally diverse individuals;

This chapter was accepted on March 23, 2006.

however, few relevant, evidence-based teaching strategies are reported in the literature. Although nursing can be transformed through the teaching of transcultural nursing (Andrews, 1995; Leininger, 1995a, 1995b; Leininger & McFarland, 2002), two major barriers prevent a rapid effective transformation. One major barrier is the lack of faculty and advanced practice nurses formally prepared in transcultural nursing and in the teaching of transcultural nursing (Andrews, 1995; Jeffreys, 2002; Leininger, 1995b). The second major barrier is the limited research evaluating the effectiveness of teaching interventions in cultural competence (Jeffreys, 2002, 2006). The future of nursing depends on the advanced development of the scholarship of teaching including theoretically and empirically supported teaching innovations (Diekelmann, 2002; Diekelmann & Ironside, 2002; Drevdahl, Stackman, Purdy, & Louie, 2002; Ironside, 2005; Jeffreys, 2004; Riley, Beal, Levi, & McCausland, 2002; Storch & Gamroth, 2002; Tanner, 2002; Young & Diekelmann, 2002). Consequently, the scholarly sharing of theoretically based teaching strategies in cultural competence education is important.

The purpose of this chapter is to describe a multidimensional strategy for teaching and learning cultural competence in graduate nursing education with a specific focus on an innovative field trip experience (IFTE). First, a brief overview of the literature in nursing and higher education provides the essential background information underlying strategy development, implementation, and evaluation, including an empirically supported conceptual model to guide cultural competence education—the Cultural Competence and Confidence (CCC) model. Next, a brief overview of the transcultural nursing core course within the Clinical Nurse Specialist (CNS) curriculum is highlighted. Four case exemplars, supplemented by detailed tables and figures, demonstrate easy application. The chapter concludes with a discussion of cognitive, practical, and affective learning outcomes and implications for nurse educators.

Background

Transcultural nursing is "a formal area of humanistic and scientific knowledge and practices focused on holistic culture care (caring) phenomena and competence to assist individuals or groups to maintain or regain their health (or well-being) and to deal with disabilities, dying, or other human conditions in culturally congruent and beneficial ways" (Leininger, 2002a, p. 84). Leininger's theory of cultural care diversity and universality, and her illustrative sunrise model (Leininger, 1991, 1994, 2002a) provide a valuable resource and guide for preparing advanced practice nurses to care for culturally diverse populations. The desired outcome of the model is cultural congruent nursing care. Culturally congruent care is care that is customized to fit with the patient's cultural values, beliefs, and practices. This requires a systematic assessment of the dynamic patterns and cultural dimensions of a particular culture (subculture or society), including religious, kinship (social), political (and legal), economic, educational, technological, and cultural values, and how these factors may be interrelated and function to influence behavior in various environmental contexts. Culturally congruent care, however, can only occur when culture care values, expressions, or patterns are known and used competently (Leininger, 2002a).

Two other frequently used conceptual frameworks include models by Campinha-Bacote (2003) and Purnell (2003). Campinha-Bacote's "Culturally Competent Model of Care" presents cultural awareness, cultural knowledge, cultural skill, cultural desire, and cultural encounters as necessary components of cultural competence. Cultural desire is introduced as the key, pivotal element in the ongoing process of cultural competence development (Campinha-Bacote, 2003). Purnell's model of cultural competence identifies areas of assessment (of clients) that will provide nurses and health care professionals with the needed information to provide cultural specific and congruent care (Purnell, 2003). The model depicts a nonlinear continuum of cultural competency ranging from the categories of unconsciously incompetent, consciously incompetent, consciously competent, and unconsciously competent. Conscious competence occurs when one seeks and obtains general knowledge about another culture, verifies generalizations about the client, and then provides culturally specific care.

These models acknowledge that cultural competency is an ongoing, complex learning process that involves continual skill acquisition and refinement. Although scholars support that all individuals, regardless of cultural background, need formalized preparation in transcultural nursing, this goal is not equally valued by all nurses (Andrews, 1995; Leininger, 1995a, 1995b; Leininger & McFarland, 2002). Because adult learners are most motivated to engage in activities that they perceive are relevant, it is important to truly capture students' interest in cultural competence development. For example, students enrolled in an adult health CNS program generally do not enter the master's program with the primary goal of developing cultural competency. "The essence of CNS practice is clinical nursing expertise in diagnosing and treatments to prevent, remediate, or alleviate illness and promote health with a defined specialty population" (NACNS, 2005, p. 5). Typically CNS students are interested in developing clinical competencies in a clinical specialty and obtaining certification in a clinical specialty; therefore, nurse educators are challenged to invigorate zeal and instill interest among these adult learners (Jeffreys, 2006).

Proponents of adult learning theory attest to the marked influence of educational enterprises, motivation, and commitment in relation to immediate career goals (Brookfield, 1986; Knowles, 1984). Adult learners will be most motivated and interested in learning if immediate benefits to career goals and daily professional responsibilities are clearly evident and learning goals are realistic. With increased globalization and the changing demographics and characteristics within and between cultural groups, it is unrealistic to expect that nurses will become specialists in caring for (or working with) all of the many different cultural groups that they may encounter.

To become a specialist in one or more select cultural groups requires a series of specialized transcultural courses and concentrated fieldwork at the graduate level (Leininger, 1989; Leininger & McFarland, 2002). It is realistic to expect that all nurses acquire the basic or generalist transcultural nursing skills needed to provide care for culturally diverse and different patients. A transcultural generalist approach emphasizes broad transcultural principles, concepts, theories, and research findings to care for patients of many different cultures (Leininger, 1989). It is also reasonable to expect that nurses who have been prepared as generalists demonstrate commitment and participate in ongoing cultural competence education. Especially pertinent are educational programs designed to expand learning with direct application to specific, targeted priority cultural groups dwelling in surrounding communities.

Despite the numerous educational opportunities available, some nurses are actively engaged in cultural competence development and direct clinical application, whereas others are not. Some nurses are more motivated to pursue cultural competence development and are more committed to the goal of culturally congruent care than others. Therefore, the consideration of factors that may influence motivation, persistence, and commitment is necessary. Confidence (self-efficacy) is one such factor (Jeffreys, 2006). According to Bandura (1986), the construct of self-efficacy is the individual's perceived confidence for learning or performing specific tasks or skills necessary to achieve a particular goal. In learning tasks, inefficacious learners are at risk for decreased motivation, lack of commitment, and/or avoidance of tasks. Learners with a resilient (strong) sense of self-efficacy in a specific domain demonstrate high levels of commitment, persistence at skill development, view difficult skills as challenges to be overcome, and expend extra energy to overcome obstacles. In contrast, supremely efficacious (overly confident) learners view tasks as insignificant and/or requiring little preparation, increasing the risk for poor outcomes. In clinical practice, avoidance of culture considerations, lack of adequate preparation, and/or rendering culturally incongruent care jeopardizes patient safety and health.

Conceptual Framework

The CCC model (Figure 2.1) demonstrates the phenomenon of learning (developing) cultural competence and incorporates the construct of transcultural self-efficacy (TSE). Transcultural self-efficacy is the perceived confidence for performing or learning general transcultural nursing skills among culturally different patients. Transcultural nursing skills are those skills necessary for assessing, planning, implementing, and evaluating culturally congruent nursing care. The performance of transcultural nursing skill competencies is directly influenced by the adequate learning of such skills and by TSE perceptions (Jeffreys, 2000, 2006).

Within the CCC model, cultural competence is defined as a multidimensional learning process that integrates transcultural skills in all three dimensions (cognitive, practical, and affective); involves TSE (confidence) as a major influencing factor; and aims to achieve culturally congruent care. The term "learning process" emphasizes that the cognitive, practical, and affective dimensions of TSE and transcultural skill development can change over time as a result of formalized education and other learning experiences. Within the context of transcultural learning, cognitive learning skills include knowledge and comprehension about ways in which cultural factors may influence professional nursing care among clients of different cultural backgrounds and throughout various

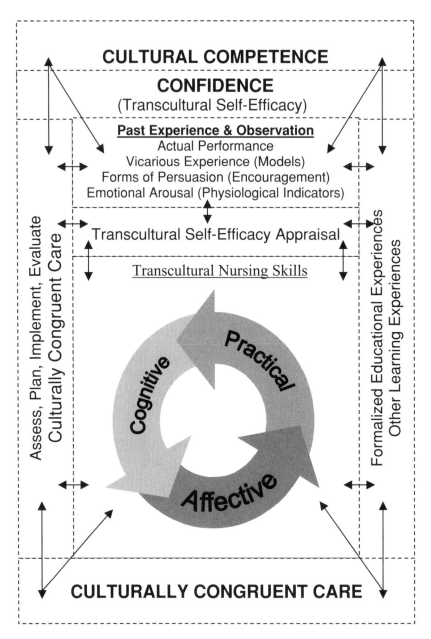

FIGURE 2.1 Jeffreys Cultural Competence and Confidence (CCC) model (2004).

Source: Jeffreys, M. R. (2006). *Teaching cultural competence in nursing and health care.* New York: Springer Publishing. Reprinted by permission.

phases of the lifecycle. The practical learning dimension is similar to the psychomotor learning domain and focuses on motor skills or practical application of skills. Within the context of transcultural learning, practical learning skills refer to communication skills (verbal and nonverbal) needed to interview clients of different cultural backgrounds about their values and beliefs. The affective learning dimension is a learning dimension concerned with attitudes, values, and beliefs and is considered to be the most important in developing professional values and attitudes. Affective learning includes self-awareness, awareness of cultural gap (differences), acceptance, appreciation, recognition, and advocacy (Jeffreys, 2006).

Formalized educational experiences and other learning experiences that (1) carefully weave cognitive, practical, and affective transcultural nursing skills; (2) encompass assessment, planning, implementation, and evaluation; and (3) integrate self-efficacy appraisals and diagnostic-specific interventions are considered essential in cultural competence education (Jeffreys, 2006). Because TSE perceptions influence a learner's actions, performance, and persistence for learning tasks associated with cultural competence development, it is important that educators fully understand the vital role of self-efficacy appraisal.

Self-efficacy appraisal is an individualized process influenced by four information sources: (1) actual performances, (2) vicarious experiences (observing role models), (3) forms of persuasion (receiving encouragement and judicious praise), and (4) emotional arousal (physiological indices). Actual performances are the strongest source of efficacy information (Bandura, 1986). Successful performances can raise efficacy, whereas unsuccessful performances lower it. Lowered self-efficacy can be psychologically stressful and dissatisfying to nurses, thereby adversely affecting motivation, persistence, and cultural competency development. Individuals with low self-efficacy initially can feel devastated by failure or poor performance, and further lowered self-efficacy can cause avoidance behaviors (Bandura, 1986, 1997). Formalized teaching strategies that provide essential background information and facilitate varied opportunities for self-directed, learner-centered interactive activities and experiential learning will be most beneficial. Combining several strategies to create empowering learning environments will promote a stronger sense of meaningfulness in task accomplishment, resilient confidence, and greater control over choices in the learning process in a truly learning-centered curricula (Candela, Dally, & Benzel-Lindley, 2006; Siu, Laschinger, & Vingilis, 2005).

Course Overview

"Transcultural Concepts and Issues in Health Care"—a 3-credit, 15-week, graduate core course within the adult health CNS curriculum—is taught at a large urban, public college that serves large numbers of various student and client cultural groups. The main aim of the course is to provide students with a strong foundation in transcultural nursing that permits purposeful integration of transcultural nursing concepts and skills at higher levels of complexity throughout the curriculum and advanced practice role development. After completion of the CNS, students may choose to pursue the nurse practitioner (NP) option.

Based on current recommendations in the literature, the course focuses on the general philosophy, ethics, concepts, skills, theory, research, and practices underlying transcultural care. Current issues in pluralism, diversity, and health care are explored in relationship to culturally competent care of advanced practitioners in multiple health care settings. Leininger's theory of Culture Care (1991) and other selected theories and research studies are critically appraised for utilization in various practice and management settings. Future directions of transcultural care are discussed, with special emphasis on advanced practice roles and how to create effectively the needed transformational changes in health care, education, practice, research, and policy. Course objectives are specifically linked to the course description, course topics, and curriculum objectives, and program outcomes. (See Jeffreys, 2002, for specific details on the transcultural course.)

Following an introduction to Leininger's theory, ethnonursing research methodology, and other conceptual models, students are introduced to various topics concerning health disparities, cultural assessment, ethnicity, race, class, gender, sexual orientation, religion, ethnopharmacology, discrimination and bias, multiple heritage individuals, female circumcision, complementary and alternative medicines, physical assessment, spirituality, and mental health. Students are expected to be active, well-prepared participants in seminar who critically discuss assigned chapters, journal articles, class films, lectures, and PowerPoint presentations. Other teaching–learning strategies involve conducting a review of the literature (ROL) on a select transcultural topic and a clinical topic (usually chosen to develop the CNS-targeted area of specialty); writing a ROL paper and connecting the ROL paper to a future CNS role; and writing a CNS paper.

Students have a choice of several CNS paper options: (1) cultural assessment enabler, (2) sphere of influence, (3) professional development: conference, (4) leadership: letter to the editor or author, or (5) IFTE. Methods of evaluation are comprised of seminar participation (30%), the ROL paper (40%), and the CNS paper (30%). The selection of multidimensional teaching and evaluation strategies are twofold: (1) to address varied learning styles among diverse learners, and (2) to stimulate learning in the cognitive, psychomotor (practical), and affective domains.

Innovative Field Trip Experience

The IFTE was a learner-centered, creative strategy that was implemented during the second half of a required transcultural core course in the CNS/NP curriculum. The IFTE included prerequisite components (background reading assignments, classroom seminar and films, literature review, and written paper); general required components (student-initiated field trip selection, purpose and objectives, instructor approval, plan, implementation, and written paper); and information-sharing/dissemination components (storytelling and cultural food buffet). Figure 2.2 presents the IFTE components as formal and informal educational experiences within the context of the CCC model.

The prerequisite components were designed to provide students with beginning foundational knowledge in transcultural nursing and in the expected role competencies of the CNS. The background reading assignments provided a common framework for seminar discussion. Films expanded on reading and prior learning, presenting students with the opportunity to gain a different perspective into the emic (insider) perspective of different cultural groups. By the third week, students selected their own review of literature topics. The process of searching the literature and available resources on both selected clinical and transcultural topics provided students with some essential "holding" knowledge. Leininger (2002b) described the powerful value of "holding" knowledge prior to interacting with members of a cultural community or

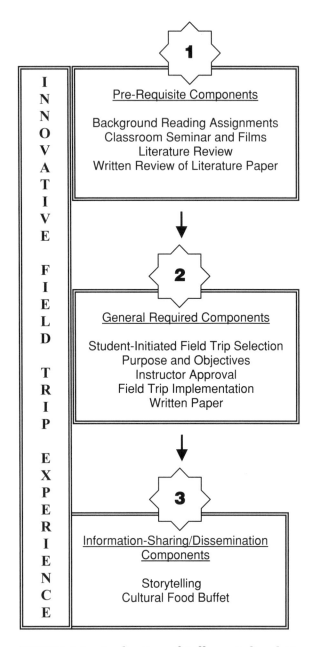

FIGURE 2.2 Application of Jeffreys Cultural Competence and Confidence model: Innovative Field Trip Experience.

engaging in other "immersion" experiences to enhance understanding of the culture.

The student's self-selection of the field trip option, formulation of purpose and objectives, and planning of the intended experience were consistent with principles of adult learning theory (Table 2.1). This process of selecting the field trip option involved reflection. When used appropriately, reflection is an effective teaching method that enhances nursing practice (Ruth-Sahd, 2003). "When students are challenged to choose topics about which they are passionate and reflect on their application of research-based evidence to clinical practice, their work reflects scholarly effort" (Sevean, Poole, & Shane Strickland, 2003, p. 475). Students must reflect on their prior learning, present stage as a learner, and future advanced practice role to create their own, individualized, and highly relevant practicum. "A reflective practicum is an experience of high interpersonal intensity. The learning predicament, the students' vulnerability, and the behavioral worlds created by coaches and students critically influence learning outcomes" (Schön, 1987, p. 171).

Although instructor approval suggested a simple dichotomous approach—the proposed field trip and objectives are approved or they are not—it was not really this simple. Within the context of adult learning theory and reflection-in-action, the role of the instructor was to guide (coach) students to further explore, shape, modify, or revise their intended experience, purposes, and/or objectives and seek a deeper level of potential learning. According to Schön (1987), professional education should be focused on enhancing the professional's ability for "reflection-in-action" or learning by doing and preparing professionals for lifelong learning and problem solving throughout professional practice. Certainly, cultural competence development involves lifelong learning, and nurse educators are in a key position to guide students.

Students' implementation of the planned field trip experience permitted further opportunity to shape the experience and engage in ongoing reflection-in-action (Table 2.2). For example, interviews, eating traditional foods, wearing traditional clothing, and other components were not preplanned, but added a valuable dimension to the experience and further enhanced cognitive, practical, and affective learning. The process of writing the CNS paper encouraged students to further reflect on and evaluate the experience and explore the connections between the field trip experience, prior learning, future learning, and application to the future CNS role. (Table 2.3). Pre-established paper grading criteria

TABLE 2.1 Topics, Field Trip Selection, and Purposes/Objectives: Comparison of Four Case Exemplars

Review of Literature Paper Title			
Promoting Prenatal Care for Asian-Indian Women through Cultural-Specific Care	Exploring Amish Cultural Beliefs and Immunization Practices	Helping Orthodox Jewish Families Cope with the End-of-Life Process in the Intensive Care Unit	Exploring Complementary and Alternative Medicines for the Management of Arthritic Pain in African-American Women
Transcultural Topic Focus			
Asian-Indian American Women	Amish culture	Orthodox Jewish community	African-American Women
Clinical Topic Focus			
Prenatal Care	Immunization beliefs and practices	End-of-life care decisions	Arthritic pain management
Reason for Interest in Topic			
Asian-Indian women have a high incidence of low birth weight infants	After gaining some general knowledge of the Amish, was intrigued to learn more	Limited knowledge in caring for the Orthodox Jew during end-of-life	Future Clinical Nurse Specialist role in pain management; Limited knowledge about African-American culture

TABLE 2.1 (*continued*)

Reason for Selecting Field Trip Experience Instead of Other Options

A chance to explore Asian-Indian culture	To fully appreciate and explore the world of the Amish in greater detail and obtain first-hand knowledge of the Amish way of life	To obtain first-hand experience and knowledge directly from members of the Orthodox Jewish community	Increase understanding of major historical and political events that shaped African-American life and culture

Name of Field Trip Selected

Deepavali festival Asian-Indian neighborhood	Amish community in Pennsylvania	Workshop on Bikur Cholim, a prescription for life (end-of-life care) held in an Orthodox Jewish high school in New York City	Exhibit on slavery in New York at a large local historical society

How Field Trip Was Selected

Association of Indians in America Web site	Review of Internet sites	Recommendation of rabbi from the work setting	Internet research

(*continued*)

TABLE 2.1 Topics, Field Trip Selection, and Purposes/Objectives: Comparison of Four Case Exemplars

Location of Field Trip			
South Street Seaport (NYC) and two Asian-Indian neighborhoods in Queens, NY	Amish community in Lancaster, Pennsylvania	New York, New York	New York, New York

Purposes/Objectives of Field Trip

1. Gain a personal experience of Asian-Indian culture 2. Gain an insider's view into Asian-Indian lifestyle 3. Gain knowledge on Asian-Indian prenatal practices	1. Gain first-hand knowledge of the Amish culture 2. Explore the Amish culture's health care beliefs 3. Gain an understanding of Amish immunization practices	1. Gain knowledge on end-of-life care of the Orthodox Jew 2. Extrapolate what health care professionals can do individually and at the institutional level to provide culturally sensitive care 3. Tap into community resources	1. Gain better understanding of African-American culture from an emic perspective 2. To corroborate the importance of spirituality and religion on African-American life 3. To acquire more background information in order to provide cultural congruent care as a Clinical Nurse Specialist

TABLE 2.2 Select Field Trip Components: Comparison of Four Case Exemplars

	Asian-Indian Women and Prenatal Care	Amish Culture and Immunization Beliefs and Practices	Orthodox Jewish Community and End-of-Life Care	African-American Women and Arthritic Pain Management Using Complementary and Alternative Medicines
Components of Field Trip	1. Deepavali festival 2. Hindu temples* 3. Asian-Indian bridal shops 4. Asian-Indian restaurant	1. Mennonite information center 2. Amish museum—dressed in Amish attire* 3. Amish farmhouse 4. Amish cuisine* 5. Amish quilt shops*	1. Workshop on "The Role of the Visitor—The How To's" 2. Workshop on "Being Present at Life's End" 3. Kosher breakfast and lunch* 4. Interviews with project manager and rabbi*	1. Historical perspective and exhibits 2. Spirituality, religion, church, and community exhibits 3. Artifacts and clothing of the era* 4. Short movies and audiotaped documentaries*
Interviewed Persons	An Asian-Indian female physician at the Deepavali festival regarding traditional health practices and implications for health professionals*	1. Woman from Mennonite Information Center* 2. Amish elderly man at the Amish farmhouse*	1. Project Manager* 2. Rabbi*	N/A

(continued)

TABLE 2.2 Select Field Trip Components: Comparison of Four Case Exemplars (*continued*)

	Asian-Indian Women and Prenatal Care	Amish Culture and Immunization Beliefs and Practices	Orthodox Jewish Community and End-of-Life Care	African-American Women and Arthritic Pain Management Using Complementary and Alternative Medicines
Interaction With Others*	Conversations with bridal shop owners and workers in two Indian neighborhoods* Worshippers in Hindu temple*	Many members of the Amish faith throughout field trip (farmhouse, quilt shops, Mennonite Center, church service)*	Workshop participants mainly comprised of Orthodox Jewish men and women in the 50- to 60-year age group. Workshops were held in semicircles and small groups to answer discussion questions of experiences with a loved one during the end-of-life and for one member to share with the group*	It was interesting to observe the different groups from various backgrounds and ages who were visiting the exhibit*
Senses Involved in the Experience*	Dance and music performances, food at the festival. Different smells and taste of spices used in food at the festival and restaurant.	Sounds of church service. Various smells at the Amish farmhouse and restaurant. Taste of different ethnic foods at restaurant. Sight and touch at museum, quilt shops, and tours.	During breakfast and lunch, the atmosphere was social and jovial, with many people greeting long-time friends and socializing	Audiotaped documentaries. Artifacts and clothing of the era were a great part of the exhibit. Cafeteria had good food and refreshments
Methods Used to Record/Remember Experience Details	Pamphlets, camera	Notes, pamphlets, photos	Notes and pamphlets	Notes, pamphlets, and newspapers

N/A, not applicable.
*Those that were not initially planned, but occurred during the field trip.

TABLE 2.3 Significance of Field Trip Experience: Comparison of Four Case Exemplars

Asian-Indian Women and Prenatal Care	Amish Culture and Immunization Beliefs and Practices	Orthodox Jewish Community and End-of-Life Care	African-American Women and Arthritic Pain Management Using Complementary and Alternative Medicines
Most Significant Component of Field Trip to ROL Paper			
Role of women in Asian-Indian culture	Personal interview with an elderly Amish man who spoke about his culture's health care beliefs and immunization practices	Recurrent themes throughout the workshop of the importance of family and community being present during end-of-life. As stated in the *Book of Genesis*, Judaism centers on the family as a unit.	Spirituality and religion are major components of African-American life, profoundly influencing health care practices and beliefs
Most Significant Component of Field Trip to Course Topics			
Visiting Deepavali festival and exploring the Asian-Indian culture	Opportunity to explore the Amish way of life experientially and speak to members of the Amish faith	One-on-one communication with members of the Orthodox Jewish community as well as authorities on the culture	To gain a sense of the hardships African Americans encountered during slavery time and how this effects the present day

(continued)

TABLE 2.3 Significance of Field Trip Experience: Comparison of Four Case Exemplars

Asian-Indian Women and Prenatal Care	Amish Culture and Immunization Beliefs and Practices	Orthodox Jewish Community and End-of-Life Care	African-American Women and Arthritic Pain Management Using Complementary and Alternative Medicines
Most Significant Component of Field Trip to Future CNS Role			
To understand the lifestyle and practices of a different culture to provide culturally appropriate care	Formulate a teaching plan to facilitate preventative health care using a culturally congruent approach	Formulate teaching plan to facilitate change at the institutional level	To provide culturally congruent care for African Americans in general as well as specialized focus on African-American women with arthritic pain
Desired Future CNS Role			
Critical care/educator	Educator	Educator in cardiac care/critical care	Pain management
Three Most Relevant CNS Competencies Further Developed Through the Field Trip			
Leadership	Research	Research	Educator
Collaboration	Leadership	Leadership	Researcher
Clinical expertise in the specialty	Collaboration	Collaboration	Partnership with faith-based centers

CNS, Clinical Nurse Specialist; ROL, review of the literature.

provided students with a common framework for focus and reflection, such as discussing the most significant field trip experience component to: (1) course topics, (2) ROL paper, (3) CNS competencies, and (4) future advanced practice role. Additionally, this aimed to validate learning via the field trip experience by demonstrating immediate and future application to the achievement of an important career goal.

The final component of the IFTE (information-sharing/dissemination through storytelling and cultural food buffet) aimed to further develop several CNS competencies: collaboration, leadership, and education, specifically within the "nurses and nursing practice" sphere of influence. Reflective storytelling was a valuable strategy that facilitated reflective analysis, enhanced self-esteem, and enriched cultural sensitivity and understanding (Davidhizar & Lonzer, 2003; Spence, 2005).

The cultural food buffet setting provided a relaxed, informal atmosphere to share stories about the ROL topic and IFTE. After reviewing Leininger's chapter concerning the cultural meaning of food (Leininger, 2002c), students took great pride in sharing traditional cultural foods (from either their own culture or researched culture) and in sharing the cultural meanings and significance of the foods. The different tastes, smells, feels, sounds, and looks of the ethnic food evoked sensory stimulation and cultural learning while also promoting positive feelings about the overall "informal presentation" experience. The brief question-and-answer session encouraged participation and dialogue between students and thereby enhanced opportunities for clarification, collaboration, education, and critical thinking. Distribution of presenters' abstracts with name and contact information provided a mechanism for ongoing networks, shared information, long-term learning, and validation.

Case Exemplars: Innovative Field Trip Experience Strategy in Action

The following actual case exemplars demonstrate application of the IFTE and present selected highlights of the learning experience from the student perspective. In addition, Tables 2.1–2.3 enhance the text by providing easy comparison among the four case exemplars: (1) Asian-Indian women and prenatal care, (2) Amish culture and immunization beliefs and practices, (3) Orthodox Jewish community and end-of-life care, and (4) African-American women and arthritic pain management using complementary and alternative medicines.

Asian-Indian Women and Prenatal Care

Concern over the prevalence of low-birth weight infants and the low rate of early prenatal care among Asian-Indian women in the United States sparked interest in further understanding the traditional cultural values, beliefs, and health care practices. Initially, the field trip plan included participant observation at a Deepavali festival. The Deepavali festival is a festival of lights that fights off the darkness in human lives; it signifies both the beginning of the Asian Indian New Year and the victory of good over evil. The celebration is spread over 1 month. Music and dancing in traditional clothing in bright colors, such as red and gold, are essential in celebrations and spiritual devotions for special occasions, because its purpose is to bring in peace and prosperity, and to keep evil and disease away.

At the festival, I (V. L.) had the opportunity to talk to a physician regarding the health practices of Asian Indians. During this informal interview and discussion, we spoke about health promotion and women's roles. In an Asian Indian family, men are the decision-makers of the family and usually make decisions for their wives. Language barrier, access to health care, and other health practices may hinder women's access to early prenatal care.

Next, the field trip expanded to include an exploration of an Asian Indian neighborhood in New York City. The neighborhood contained many bridal shops, because weddings are big occasions in the Asian Indian community. As I was visiting the various bridal shops, I thought of the idea that prenatal teaching should be made available here, because it is a place where future brides would visit. Because the majority of Asian Indians are Hindu, I also visited two Hindu temples. I learned that before entering the temples, I needed to remove my shoes and place them on the shoe racks located outside. Because Hindu temples are places of worship, shoe racks are placed outside for worshippers to take off their shoes before entering. Shoes are viewed as unclean, and cleanliness must be preserved within the temple.

The field trip enabled me to gain a personal experience of Asian-Indian culture, gain an insider's view into Asian-Indian lifestyle, and gain knowledge about Asian-Indian prenatal practices. Through the various components of the field trip experience, I further developed competencies in collaboration, leadership, and clinical expertise. By further understanding the lifestyle and practices of a different culture, I will be better prepared to provide culturally appropriate care. Future potential networks include collaboration with physicians within the cultural community and proactively providing women's health teaching through cooperative alliances at bridal shops.

Amish Culture and Immunization Beliefs and Practices

Recent concerns over the outbreak of infectious disease occurring in Amish communities first prompted a ROL about the Amish and immunization practices. The desire to appreciate and explore the world of the Amish in greater detail and obtain first-hand knowledge about the Amish culture, particularly immunization practices and health care beliefs, inspired an overnight trip to Lancaster, Pennsylvania. To accomplish these objectives, the following visits were planned: Mennonite Information Center, tour of a functional Amish farmhouse, driving tours, and the Lancaster County History Museum. The most powerful sensory experiences of the trip were the:

- lull of streets without automobiles,
- clear sky missing the chaos of telephone lines,
- sweet smell of wheat and tobacco fields,
- heavy taste of shoo fly pie, and
- soft feel of handmade quilts skillfully crafted by the community over many hours juxtaposed to the stiff, constricting feel that I experienced when dressed in traditional Amish attire.

Although not originally planned, my (L. B.) personal interviews with a woman from the Mennonite Center and an elderly Amish man at the farmhouse proved to be the most significant and compelling component of the trip. As we conversed, they enlightened me about the constant need to relate cultural beliefs, values, and customs to nursing practice. For example, the Amish man spoke about his culture's health care beliefs and immunization practices. Through a personal interview with the Amish man, I was provided with the fundamental framework on why and how Amish immunization practices are upheld. To my surprise, I learned that a major factor of under-immunization is financial—most

Amish people do not receive immunizations because they are too costly for the whole family.

Furthermore, in relation to the Amish striving for autonomy, I discovered that when the state of Pennsylvania announced that immunizations would be provided free of charge, church bishops informed the Amish community that this would be accepting charity from the modern world, an unacceptable action. Although the church does not restrict immunizations, it is not a recommended practice; church leaders greatly influence health practice within the community. As a future CNS within the desired educator role, the field trip experience will assist me formulating a teaching plan to facilitate preventive health care using a culturally congruent approach.

Orthodox Jewish Community and End-of-Life Care

Providing culturally competent end-of-life care for Orthodox Jewish patients and their families first required an in-depth comprehension of Orthodox Jewish values and beliefs. Based on my (J. D.) hospital rabbi's recommendation, participation at a Bikur Cholim (visiting the sick) workshop was ideal. The experience gave me an in-depth understanding of the roles and responsibilities of the Orthodox Jewish community when a member of the community is sick or dying.

Although initial objectives targeted workshop attendance and information gathering, other learning and networking opportunities emerged. Through workshop attendance, contacts were made with professionals in the Orthodox Jewish community who had programs in place for meeting their community's end-of-life needs. These programs could be helpful blueprints that health care professionals can adapt and incorporate into their plan of care when working with the Orthodox Jewish community during end-of-life. Future networking can provide links to assist nurses, other health professionals, and organizations in planning and providing culturally specific care to Orthodox Jews.

African-American Women and Arthritic Pain Management Using Complementary and Alternative Medicines

Pain perception and pain management involve highly personalized experiences that are greatly influenced by culture. My (S. N.) broad aim was to learn more about African-American women and arthritic pain management using complementary and alternative medicine. I recognized that the choice and use of complementary and alternative medicines and Western medicine options are often influenced by ethnohistorical, social, and political factors, especially among minority groups historically suffering discrimination and oppression. The "Slavery in New York" exhibit at the local historical society provided a unique opportunity to gain further insight. The exhibit gave a great understanding of the major events that shaped African-American women's life and culture.

Consistent with my ROL, the church proved once more to be the center of life for African Americans and a trusted social network. I learned that despite all adversities these women encountered, they shared "a community invisible to most whites, meeting secretly, burying their dead with dignity and preserving traces of Africa" (museum exhibit statement by Professor James Oliver Horton, chief historian, 2005). Today, many African-American churches have become quite structured, with leaders who can influence every aspect of life. Although churches are not traditional health care settings, faith communities have been long involved in providing health care.

The field trip gave me a deeper understanding of African-American culture and helped me identify the elements that will make a difference in providing culturally congruent care for these clients. As evidenced in the museum exhibits, pamphlets, and other literature, African Americans apply their religious and spiritual beliefs and practices to cope with some of life's most challenging circumstances. Church, spirituality, and prayer were found to be the factors that profoundly influence health care practices and beliefs of African-American women. I realized that the CNS should attempt to work in a partnership with faith-based centers to enhance health promotion and provide health education for African Americans on how to cope with chronic diseases and symptoms, such as arthritic pain. The CNS can also improve quality of care by gaining cultural-specific knowledge and by disseminating information and research findings to nurses, other health professionals, and health care organizations.

Learning Outcomes

Evaluation of a multidimensional teaching strategy involves a multidimensional evaluation plan that assesses cognitive, practical, and affective learning. To systematically appraise learning outcomes for presentation in this chapter, students completed surveys about their perceived learning outcomes as a result of the field trip experiences described in this chapter. The instructor adapted a learning outcome survey from the Transcultural Self-Efficacy Tool (Jeffreys, 1994, 2006). To evaluate different levels of cognitive learning outcomes, students were first asked whether they gained new knowledge, comprehended knowledge better, learned to apply knowledge, learned how to analyze information differently, or learned how to synthesize (repattern) information differently for a selection of 53 items. Next, to evaluate practical learning, students identified interview topics among the same 53 items. Formal interviews or conversations with people within the specific culture were included. Finally, affective learning outcomes were assessed by asking students whether they gained new or further developed existing attitudes, values, or beliefs concerning 30 items.

Although self-report findings must be viewed cautiously, evaluation of cultural competence behaviors in the clinical setting would be difficult. Self-report measures provide valuable insight into the student experience, perceptions of learning, and confidence (self-efficacy)—factors that influence cultural competence development and provision of culturally congruent care; therefore, further discussion is justified. As anticipated, student cognitive and practical learning outcomes were varied, based on topics and setting. For example, only one student reported comprehension about "life support and resuscitation;" this student's field trip concerned end-of-life issues for Orthodox Jewish patients. In contrast, all students reported cognitive learning for "religious background and identity," "religious practices and beliefs," and "traditional health and illness beliefs."

Comparison of perceived cognitive, practical, and affective learning outcomes identified several interesting findings:

- All students reported cognitive and affective learning outcomes.
- The three participatory-observation experiences resulted in cognitive, practical, and affective learning outcomes; these experiences involved direct interaction and interview with informants within the selected culture.
- The observation-only field trip (museum experience) resulted in the highest number of cognitive learning items.

- Cognitive learning occurred mainly on knowledge and comprehension levels.
- About members of different cultural groups, all students reported affective learning outcomes across several categories: awareness, acceptance, appreciation, recognition, and advocacy.

Implications for Nurse Educators

The literature reveals an alarming gap in conceptually and empirically supported teaching strategies, especially those targeting cultural competence development within clinically focused graduate nursing programs. Furthermore, teaching strategies designed to address the holistic learner—incorporating cognitive, practical (psychomotor), and affective skills—are grossly underrepresented in the literature. The IFTE is a learner-centered, creative strategy that involves a carefully orchestrated integration of cognitive, practical, and affective skills. Implemented during the second half of a required transcultural core course in the CNS/NP curriculum, the IFTE assisted beginning graduate students to enrich their cultural competence; gain insight into the emic (insider) perspective; and develop clinical expertise through formalized and informal, self-directed educational experiences. Positive student responses for the IFTE, as well as positive learner outcomes, support its continued use. The four case exemplars demonstrate easy application for use in various settings, list methods to evaluate learning, and identify learning outcomes achieved.

Future empirical investigation of the IFTE, adapted to various student populations and settings, are recommended. To expand the repertoire of conceptually and empirically supported teaching strategies, nurse educators must exert an active role in the scholarship of teaching, participate in the ongoing dissemination of educational scholarship, challenge the status quo when appropriate, advocate for positive change, and replace teacher-centered pedagogy with learner-centered approaches.

REFERENCES

Andrews, M. (1995). Transcultural nursing: Transforming the curriculum. *Journal of Transcultural Nursing, 6*(2), 4–9.

Bandura, A. (1986). *Social foundations of thought and action: A social cognitive theory.* Englewood Cliffs, NJ: Prentice-Hall.

Bandura, A. (1997). *Self-efficacy: The exercise of control.* New York, NY: W.H. Freeman.

Brookfield, S.D. (1986). *Understanding and facilitating adult learning.* San Francisco, CA: Jossey-Bass.

Campinha-Bacote, J. (2003). *The process of cultural competence in the delivery of healthcare services: A culturally competent model of care* (4th ed.). Cincinnati, OH: Transcultural C.A.R.E. Associates.

Candela, L., Dalley, K., & Benzel-Lindley, J. (2006). A case for learning-centered curricula. *Journal of Nursing Education, 45,* 59–68.

Davidhizar, R., & Lonser, G. (2003). Storytelling as a teaching technique. *Nurse Educator, 28,* 217–221.

Diekelmann, N. (2002). "She asked this simple question": Reflecting and the scholarship of teaching. *Journal of Nursing Education, 41,* 381–382.

Diekelmann, N., & Ironside, P. M. (2002). Developing a science of nursing education: Innovation with research. *Journal of Nursing Education, 41,* 379–380.

Drevdahl, D. J., Stackman, R. W., Purdy, J. M., & Louie, B. Y. (2002). Merging reflective inquiry and self-study as a framework for enhancing the scholarship of teaching. *Journal of Nursing Education, 41,* 413–418.

Horton, J. O. (2005). *Slavery in New York* (exhibit). New York Historical Society, New York, New York.

Ironside, P. M. (2005). Teaching thinking and reaching the limits of memorization: Enacting new pedagogies. *Journal of Nursing Education, 44,* 441–449.

Jeffreys, M. R. (1994). *Transcultural self-efficacy tool (TSET).* Unpublished instrument copyrighted by author.

Jeffreys, M. R. (2000). Development and psychometric evaluation of the Transcultural Self-Efficacy Tool: A synthesis of findings. *Journal of Nursing Education, 11,* 127–136.

Jeffreys, M. R. (2002). A transcultural core course in the clinical nurse specialist curriculum. *Clinical Nurse Specialist: The Journal for Advanced Nursing Practice, 16*(4), 195–202.

Jeffreys, M. R. (2004). *Nursing student retention: Understanding the process and making a difference.* New York: Springer Publishing.

Jeffreys, M. R. (2005). Clinical nurse specialists as cultural brokers, change agents, and partners in meeting the needs of culturally diverse populations. *Journal of Multicultural Nursing and Health, 11*(2), 41–48.

Jeffreys, M. R. (2006). *Teaching cultural competence in nursing and health care: Inquiry, action, and innovation.* New York: Springer Publishing.

Knowles, M. (1984). *The adult learner: A neglected species.* Houston, TX: Gulf.

Leininger, M. M. (1989). Transcultural nurse specialists and generalists: New practitioners in nursing. *Journal of Transcultural Nursing, 1,* 4–16.

Leininger, M. M. (1991). *Culture care diversity and universality: A theory of nursing.* New York, NY: National League for Nursing.

Leininger, M. M. (1994). *Transcultural nursing: Concepts, theories, and practices.* Columbus, OH: Greyden Press.

Leininger, M. M. (1995a). *Transcultural nursing: Concepts, theories, research, and practice.* Blacklick, OH: McGraw-Hill College Custom Services.

Leininger, M. M. (1995b). Teaching transcultural nursing in undergraduate and graduate programs. *Journal of Transcultural Nursing, 6*(2), 10–26.

Leininger, M. M. (2002a). Part I: The theory of culture care. In M. M. Leininger & M. R. McFarland (Eds.), *Transcultural nursing: Concepts, theories, research, and practice* (3rd ed., pp. 71–98). New York, NY: McGraw-Hill.

Leininger, M. M. (2002b). Transcultural nursing and globalization of health care: Importance, focus, and historical aspects. In M. M. Leininger & M. R. McFarland (Eds.), *Transcultural nursing: Concepts, theories, research, and practice* (3rd ed., pp. 3–43). New York, NY: McGraw-Hill.

Leininger, M. M. (2002c). Transcultural food functions, beliefs, and practices. In M. M. Leininger & M. R. McFarland (Eds.), *Transcultural nursing: Concepts, theories, research, and practice* (3rd ed., pp. 205–216). New York, NY: McGraw-Hill.

Leininger, M. M., & McFarland, M. R. (2002). *Transcultural nursing: Concepts, theories, research, and practice* (3rd ed.). New York, NY: McGraw-Hill.

National Association of Clinical Nurse Specialists (NACNS). (2005). *Statement on clinical nurse specialist practice and education.* Glenview, IL: National Association of Clinical Nurse Specialists.

Purnell, L. D. (2003). Purnell's model for cultural competence. In L. D. Purnell & B. J. Paulanka (Eds.), *Transcultural health care: A culturally competent approach* (2nd ed., pp. 8–39). Philadelphia: F.A. Davis.

Riley, J. M., Beal, J., Levi, P., & McCausland, M. P. (2002). Revisioning nursing scholarship. *Journal of Nursing Scholarship, 34*(4), 383–389.

Ruth-Sahd, L. A. (2003). Reflective practice: A critical analysis of data-based studies and implications for nursing education. *Journal of Nursing Education, 42,* 488–497.

Schön, D. (1987). *Educating the reflective practitioner.* San Franscisco, CA: Jossey-Bass.

Sevean, P. A., Poole, K., & Shane Strickland, D. (2005). Actualizing scholarship in senior baccalaureate students. *Journal of Nursing Education, 44,* 473–476.

Siu, H. M., Laschinger, H. K., & Vingilis, E. (2005). The effect of problem-based learning on nursing students' perceptions of empowerment. *Journal of Nursing Education, 44,* 459–469.

Spence, D. G. (2005). Hermeneutic notions augment cultural safety education. *Journal of Nursing Education, 44,* 409–414.

Storch, J., & Gamroth, L. (2002). Scholarship revisited: A collaborative nursing education program's journey. *Journal of Nursing Education, 41*(2), 524–530.

Tanner, C. A. (2002). Learning to teach: An introduction to "Teacher talk: New pedagogies for nursing." *Journal of Nursing Education, 41*(3), 95–96.

Young, P., & Diekelmann, N. (2002). Learning to lecture: Exploring the skills, strategies, and practices of new teachers in nursing education. *Journal of Nursing Education, 41*(9), 405–412.

Chapter 3

Providing Time Out: A Unique Service Learning Clinical Experience

Jayne Kendle and Linda H. Zoeller

When their triplets were born at 26 weeks gestation, Casey and Bob entered the world of parenting medically fragile children. They were overwhelmed. When the babies were discharged, the family's home took on the appearance of an intensive care unit with monitors, oxygen canisters, tubing, feeding pumps, and various other medical supplies. Lily and Chad required oxygen therapy, breathing treatments, and nasogastric tube feedings every 3 hours. Michael had a tracheostomy, was fed via a gastrostomy tube (G-tube), and required multiple medications and breathing treatments throughout the day and night.

The family's income was cut in half when Casey realized she would not be able to return to work. Casey was relieved when it was determined that Bob's insurance would provide 8 hours of nursing care/day for Michael while Bob was at work, but the couple had no assistance in the evenings, at night, or on weekends. Their sense of being overwhelmed was soon replaced by utter exhaustion. After months of sleepless nights, the couple saw no "light at the end of the tunnel." Fatigue changed the dynamics of the couple's communication. Fights followed by stony silences became the norm. Casey became depressed, fearing that her family was falling apart, and there was no place to go for help.

This chapter was accepted on March 23, 2006.

This chapter illustrates one approach to addressing the community need for pediatric respite care while meeting the learning needs of nursing students.

A Growing Population

Casey and Bob's situation is not unique. Advances in perinatology, neonatology, and pediatric care have resulted in a growing population of families raising medically fragile, technology-dependent and/or developmentally delayed children (Miller, 2002; Olsen & Maslin-Prothero, 2001; Robinson, Jackson, & Townsley, 2001). Although the general consensus is that the population of children with special needs is growing, the extent of this population is unknown. There is no system in place that tracks the actual number of children with special needs or the degree to which the special need affects the child and family. This lack of reporting contributes directly to the public's lack of understanding of the needs of families with these children.

Effects of Chronic Caregiving on Family Members

Although the ultimate goal of nurses and physicians working with ill neonates and children is to discharge the child to their home, few professionals realize how the lives of the parent(s), sibling(s), and extended family can change when a child is discharged with chronic complications. The life stories of families with children with special needs are inspiring yet tragic. These parents devote their lives to caring for their children in ways that go above and beyond what typical parenting requires. Caregiving for these parents often entails hours of physical care and therapies. They frequently go days, weeks, or even months at a time without an uninterrupted night sleep. They live with uncertainty, never knowing what tomorrow will bring. The risk that serious illness (or possibly death) is right around the corner for their child is a daily reality (Sokol, 1995). Unfortunately, the work of these parents is often invisible to professionals, policy makers, and the general public as the parents struggle at home, in silence, to care for their child (Ray, 2002).

The toll that chronic caregiving has on the primary caregiver, the marriage, and other children has been studied (Baum, 2004; Harrigan, Ratliffe, Patrinos, & Tse, 2002; Miller, 2002; Montagnino & Mauricio,

2004; Thurgate, 2005; Withers & Bennett, 2003). Mothers of medically fragile children often assume the majority of the responsibility for the day-to-day care of their children (Valkenier, Hayes, & McElheran, 2002). These mothers have been shown to have increased rates of depression, decreased rates of overall health, less family support, and fewer opportunities for recreational and cultural activities than mothers of similar age children without disabilities (Thyen, Terres, Yazdgerdi, & Perrin, 1998). Mothers often report being "worn out" by the care of their child. Major concerns of fathers of medically fragile children have been reported to include having enough money to meet family needs and the inability to get out of the house and have quality time alone with their spouse (Heaman, 1995).

In a study by Ray (2002), parents described being tired and approaching "burn out." Parents frequently reported a strong sense of isolation and inconsistent support from family, neighbors, and friends. With their time and energy consumed in caring for their "sick" child, parents are unable to meet their own needs and those of other children in the family.

Studies on the impact of chronic caregiving on family members have come to the same conclusion: families caring for medically fragile, technology-dependent and/or developmentally delayed children need respite care. Respite care is a supportive service that allows families with children with special needs to take a break from the constant vigilance required to care for their children. Benefits of respite services extend beyond the parent and child with special needs to the entire family, allowing the family time to be "normal." Whereas many governmental agencies and health care professionals view respite care as "supplemental," parents view respite care as vital to the function of the family. This disparity in understanding may be because those medically fragile, technology-dependent, and/or developmentally delayed children are cared for in the home and thus remain hidden from community profiling (Folden & Coffman, 1993; MacDonald & Callery, 2004; Parra, 2003; Thurgate, 2005).

Service Learning

The concept of service learning is not new. The idea of education with a community focus has come in and out of vogue for more than 100 years.

In the United States, there was an increased interest in service learning associated with the student community activism of the 1960s and 1970s. By the late 1970s, service learning programs were on the decline as a result of decreased financial support and weak pedagogical underpinnings (Bailey, Carpenter, & Harrington, 1999). The current impetus for the growth of service learning in higher education has been, in part, a response to policy of the Higher Learning Commission (2003). One of their accreditation criteria, engagement and service, requires that the educational institution identifies its constituencies and serves them in ways that both parties value. In their 1999 position statement, *Nursing Education's Agenda for the 21st Century*, the American Association of Colleges of Nursing (AACN) declared that the evolution of nursing requires greater linkage among teaching, community service, practice, research, and the external environment (AACN, 1999).

There are numerous definitions of service learning offered in the literature. Although there are some variations within these definitions, they tend to include the following common characteristics:

- community needs are met through the service provided
- students learn and develop through active participation and reflection
- service is integrated into the academic curriculum
- civic responsibility is encouraged
- students use newly acquired skills and knowledge in real-life situations
- the development of a sense of caring for others and intangible values, such as empathy and social responsibility, are fostered (Bailey et al., 2002; Garth, Felicitti, & Sigmon, 2004; Peterson & Schaffer, 2001; Rogers, 2001; Seifer & Vaughn, 2002; Weingarten, 2003).

In many schools of nursing, service learning is a component of a community health nursing course. However, as nursing program enrollments increase and there are more nursing students than there are in-hospital clinical placements, it is becoming necessary for other nursing courses to look to the community to assist in meeting the learning needs of their students. The program outlined in this chapter is an example of a service learning program that is an integral part of a pediatric nursing course.

Pediatric Respite Care as a Service Learning Clinical Experience

Over the past 4 decades, the caring environment for children with special needs has shifted from institutions to the home. This shift in the caring environment resulted from cost containment policies, new medical technologies, and a humanitarian philosophy advocating home as the "least restrictive" environment for children (Brust, Leonard, & Sielaff, 1992; Parish, Pomeranz, Hemp, Rizzolo, & Braddock, 2001).

Multiple articles have been published documenting the need for respite services for families with children with special needs (Ashworth & Baker, 2000; Baumgardner & Burtea, 1998; Neufeld, Query, & Drummond, 2001; Thyen, Terres, Yazdgerdi, & Perrin, 1998; Treneman, Corkery, Dowdney, & Hammond, 1997). However, there continues to be a sobering lack of services and alternatives available for these families. Federal and state funds to support the care of children with special needs (including funds for respite care) continue to be decreased.

Standards related to the granting of Medicaid and Medicaid waivers to assist families are complex and vary from state to state (Cernoch, 1992; McManus et al., n.d.; Parish et al., 2001). In Indiana, for example, the waiting list for Medicaid waivers (which can financially support respite care) is 3–4 years. Once Medicaid waivers are granted, there is no guarantee that respite providers will be available. After waiting for 3 years, one local mother received a letter from the state government stating that her son had been awarded a Medicaid waiver. The letter went on to assure her that she could realistically expect to start receiving respite services in 10 years (because of a shortage in caregivers). The mother stated she did not know whether she should laugh or cry when she read the letter.

Nursing students are an untapped resource that could provide some relief for families with children with special needs. Nursing students have the basic education necessary to care for most children with special needs living in the community. They have cardiopulmonary resuscitation (CPR) training and are educated in assessment, basic nursing skills (e.g., tube feedings), childhood development, and family theory. Their education makes nursing students uniquely prepared to work with families in a service learning cooperative. For these reasons, the pediatric faculty of Saint Mary's College developed a pediatric respite program called Time Out. All nursing students enrolled in pediatric nursing participate in this program as part of their clinical experience.

Program Objectives

The primary goal of the Time Out Pediatric Respite Care experience is to allow the student to develop a professional relationship with a family that has a child with special needs. When nurses care for a sick child, they are (by the nature of the dependency of the child on the family) also caring for a sick family. Being in the home with a family allows the student to experience the impact that a child's chronic illness has on all members of the family. In the home environment, it is natural for the student to see the parent as the expert regarding his/her child. This is a paradigm shift from what the student experiences in the hospital where the physicians and nurse are often viewed as the "expert."

The respite experience makes the concept of "family-centered care" a reality for the student. Students learn from the parents, siblings, and from the child with special needs. By enhancing the students' understanding of the effects of chronicity on the family, it is believed that the student (and future nurse) will be more effective when providing care to all of their patients and their family caregivers. The nurse will know to listen to the family and to appreciate the family's input into the care of their loved one. This is a perspective that most families with chronically ill children find lacking when they interact with nurses in acute care settings (Godshall, 2003).

Program History

The Time Out Pediatric Respite Care program was initially started as a cooperative effort between Saint Mary's College and Sacred Heart Parish (Notre Dame, Indiana). Sacred Heart Parish started a geriatric respite program in 1995. Their program provided respite services primarily for family caregivers of infirmed elderly. As word of the Sacred Heart program spread through the community, the Sacred Heart parish nurses began receiving requests for pediatric respite services. Recognizing the community's need for such services and the parish's inability to meet that need, the parish nurse approached Saint Mary's College Department of Nursing to determine if the nursing program could help.

The parish nurse and the child health nursing faculty worked collaboratively to develop guidelines for a pediatric respite clinical placement. A pilot program using nursing students to provide respite care for families began in the spring of 1998 (Kendle & Campanale, 2001). When changes in the parish nurse position occurred in 2001, the pediatric respite program became the sole responsibility of the pediatric nursing faculty of Saint Mary's College.

Program Referrals

The families who initially contacted the parish nurse were the first families to participate in the Time Out respite program. As awareness of the program spread through the community, program referrals started coming from the local neonatal intensive care unit, pediatric unit, and pediatric intensive care unit nurses and social workers, First Steps Coordinators, and occupational therapists. In addition, families continue to contact the program coordinator directly after hearing about the program through friends or family support groups.

Program Guidelines

There are currently 40 families enrolled in the respite program. The ages of the children enrolled range from 6 months to 13 years. The degree of disability of the participating children varies from subtle to severe. Many of the children have varying degrees of cerebral palsy; several have seizure disorders and/or are fed via G-tubes. One child requires continuous positive airway pressure, two children have tracheostomies, and many more require suctioning and breathing treatments on a regular basis. Figure 3.1 shows one of the children in our program. Many of the children have sensory deficits, the most common being an inability to verbally communicate.

Because of the wide variety of variables that affect the family's ability to cope with the demands of caring for a child with special needs, it is difficult to draw the line related to who qualifies for the program and who does not. Essentially, the criteria for inclusion into the program is the child's "special need" prohibits the parent(s) from using the "kid next door" to baby-sit.

Guidelines that direct the respite experience have been developed and refined over the past 8 years. Initially, the students were not allowed to administer tube feedings or any type of medications. Parent evaluation

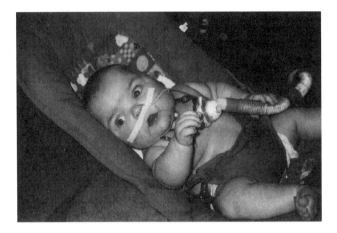

FIGURE 3.1   One of the children students are caring for in their clinical experience.
Source: Reprinted by permission, February 25, 2006.

of those guidelines reflected that this limited the benefits of the respite program because parents found it difficult to schedule activities around all feedings and medication times. Early program modifications allowed the students to administer feedings. With the addition of the waiver of liability, the students were allowed to administer medications with parental approval. Parents and students have been appreciative of the program modifications. The parents were given more flexibility, and the students felt that they were truly helping the families while gaining additional clinical nursing experience.

Program Guidelines for Families

To participate in the Time Out Pediatric Respite Care Program, parents must read and complete a waiver of liability (Figure 3.2) and a registration sheet (Figure 3.3). The registration sheet is printed on bright pink paper (commonly referred to as "the pink sheet"), which makes it easy for the family and student to find. These forms are sent to the parents to complete when they request services from the program. After the completed forms are returned to the program coordinator, the information

WAIVER OF LIABILITY AND HOLD HARMLESS AGREEMENT

This is a legal document, which includes a release of liability. Read it carefully before signing it.

1. I desire to participate in the Time Out Pediatric Respite Care through Saint Mary's College.
2. I understand my participation in the activity is totally voluntary.
3. I specifically and completely release, hold harmless, and indemnify Saint Mary's College, Notre Dame, Indiana, and all of their officers, employees, and agents (RELEASEES) from all liability, including negligence, and other causes of action, debts, claims, and demands of every kind which I have now or which may arise out of or in connection with my participation in this activity.
4. It is my express intent that this Agreement shall bind the members of my family and spouse, if I am alive, and my heirs, assigns, and personal representative, if I am deceased, and shall be deemed as a RELEASE, WAIVER, DISCHARGE AND COVENANT NOT TO SUE the above named RELEASEES. I hereby further agree that this Waiver of Liability and Hold Harmless Agreement shall be construed in accordance with the laws of the State of Indiana.
5. I further agree to release, indemnify and hold harmless the RELEASEES above from any claim, loss, liability, damage or cost, including attorney fees that they may incur due to my participation in this activity.
6. I have read this Agreement, understand its terms, have had an opportunity to consult with legal counsel and therefore now execute it voluntarily and with full knowledge of its significance.
7. I give permission for the student respite provider to administer routine and/or scheduled medications to my child._____ (Initial here)
8. I do not give permission for the student respite provider to administer routine and/or scheduled medications to my child._____ (Initial here)

Required Signatures:

Date: _____   _____
                          Signature of Participant

                          _____
                          Signature of Parent or Legal Guardian

Emergency Information:
Contact: _____
          Print Name   Relationship
Home Phone _____   Work Phone _____

FIGURE 3.2   Waiver of liability.

Source: Reprinted by permission of Rita Weiss, RPh, JD, March 14, 2006.

Time Out Pediatric Respite Care
Registration Sheet

Child's Name: _____ Date of Birth: _____

Parent(s) Name(s): _____

Siblings: Name/DOB:_____

        Will sibling(s) be at home when respite care is provided? Yes / No

Address: _____

_____

Phone Numbers: Home: _____ Cell: _____

                  Other: _____

E-mail address:_____

Child's Primary Medical Diagnoses/Health Care Problems:

_____

_____

In case of emergency:

Hospital preference: (circle one)

Memorial Hospital/Saint Joseph Regional Medical Center/other _____

MEDICATIONS your child is currently taking: (add an additional sheet if necessary)

Medication Name   Times of Administration   Special Instructions

SEIZURES: Does your child have seizures? Yes / No

If yes, describe his/her "typical" seizure: _____

_____

_____

How long does his/her seizure usually last? _____

What should the student do for your child if he/she has a seizure? (what do you usually do when your child has a seizure?)_____

_____

If the seizure lasts longer than _____ minutes, the students should call 911.

BREATHING: Does your child have asthma/breathing difficulties? Yes / No

If yes, does your child receive home breathing treatments? Yes/No

If yes, what medication(s) does your child receive/how often? _____

Special instructions related to breathing (ex. Oxygen use, suctioning) _____

_____

_____

FIGURE 3.3   Registration form.

FEEDINGS:

Does your child have a g-tube? Yes/No

     If yes, does his/her feeding go in by gravity or pump? (circle one)

     How long should the feeding be administered over? _____

     Does your child have reflux? Yes/No

     If yes, how long after a feeding before you can lay your child flat? _____

Does your child have any special feeding instructions? Yes/ No

     If yes, please describe: _____

     _____

     _____

TOILETING:

Does your child use the toilet? Yes/No

     If yes, how often should he/she be encouraged to use the toilet?_____

     If no, how often should he/she be changed?_____

     Please describe any special instructions related to toileting/skin care of the diaper area: ___

     _____

     _____

ACTIVITY/MOBILITY: Please describe any special care required related to activity.

     (Including: How often do you reposition your child? Does you child wear any special braces
or orthotics? If so, how often are they removed & replaced? What activities does your child
enjoy?) _____

     _____

     _____

     _____

     _____

ADDITIONAL INSTRUCTIONS:_____

_____

_____

_____

_____

Please contact the Time Out Program Coordinator if you have any problems with the respite care
you are provided, or if you have suggestions to improve the program.

Office phone: _____

Home phone: _____

Cell phone: _____

Email: _____

Address:_____

     _____

     _____

Respite Care Provider/phone number(s)/email address:

_____

FIGURE 3.3 (*continued*)

is entered onto a "master" copy of the form that can be printed off each semester. The program coordinator clarifies/updates the information on the registration forms with the parents every semester.

Although it is preferred that the parents administer any medications prior to or after the respite visit, student respite care providers may administer medications if the parents prepare and label the medicine in advance. Any special instructions related to the medication administration must be written down for the student respite care provider. For example, one child in the program is on Reglan. Before leaving their house, the parent draws the medication up, labels it, and leaves a note to "Give the Reglan 30 minutes before the 2 p.m. feeding." Another child suffers from grand mal seizures. His instruction sheet reads "Administer the prefilled syringe of rectal diastat (in refrigerator) if seizure lasts longer than 10 minutes."

Each parent is responsible for orienting the student respite care provider to all equipment and procedures that they will be required to perform, such as G-tube feedings, respiratory treatments, and suctioning equipment (Figure 3.4). The parent is also responsible for leaving

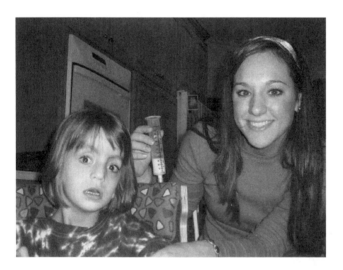

FIGURE 3.4   Parents are responsible for orienting students to equipment and procedures that their child needs during the experience.
Source: Reprinted by permission, February 25, 2006.

detailed instructions outlining the care required by their child. For example, one parent left a note for the student stating, "Molly's 10 a.m. feeding was late today. Please start her next feeding 30 minutes later than usual. This will gradually get her back on schedule." The parent must also leave emergency phone numbers and a completed pink sheet prominently displayed for the student's reference.

Parents are reminded each semester that their respite provider is a student nurse. Although students have current CPR certification and basic assessment skills, in the event of an emergency the only expectation of student performance is that they recognize that the child is in distress and call 911.

Program Guidelines for Students

Each student is required to provide 16 hours of respite care to his/her assigned family. This represents about 20% of the students' pediatric clinical experience. It is required that each student provides a minimum of 2 hours per respite visit so that the parent(s) can plan activities for themselves or with other family members. Respite visits typically last 3–4 hours. It is stressed with each student that if the respite experience is to be beneficial to the family, scheduling must be a cooperative effort between the family and student (Figure 3.5).

During the first week of the semester, students enrolled in the child health nursing course are oriented to the respite program. At this time, program objectives and program expectations are reviewed. The families enrolled in the program are discussed with the entire class. The age and special needs of each child are provided, as well as the number/ages of siblings. Family preferences related to the timing of respite services are also shared. Students have 2 days to consider which family they would like to work with. A sign-up sheet is posted that identifies the family only by the child's first name and diagnosis. The sign-up process for respite families is based on a first come, first served model.

After selecting a family, every student is accompanied by the course faculty for an introductory visit. The purpose of the first visit is for the student to learn how to get to the family's home and to meet members of the household, including the child with special needs. The visit also allows the faculty an opportunity to catch up on how the child/family has been doing since the last visit and to update the pink sheet.

SAINT MARY' S COLLEGE
DEPARTMENT OF NURSING
N326 CHILD HEALTH NURSING

STUDENT GUIDELINES FOR PEDIATRIC RESPITE PROGRAM

1.   Each student must provide 16 hours (minimum) of respite for their assigned client/family.

2.   The student should plan to spend a minimum of 2 hours per visit with their respite child. (This can be negotiated with the respite family to better meet their needs).

3.   **UNDER NO CIRCUMSTANCES** are students allowed to transport the child and/or family in the students' own vehicles.

4.   Students may (if they choose) accompany the child/family to one (or more) of the child's therapies but they must provide their own transportation. Students **ARE NOT** allowed to ride in the respite family's vehicle.

5.   The student **MUST** complete a medication sheet for all of the medications that their child is taking. Each medication sheet must be reviewed by N326 course faculty prior to the first respite visit. This sheet will be kept in the home (stapled to the pink sheet) for student reference. All med sheets will be turned in at the end of the semester.

6.   Students are **discouraged** from administering any form of medicine to their assigned respite child. **The student can only administer medications that the parent has prepared and labeled. Any special instructions related to the medication and its administration must be written down by the parents for the student.**

7.   After completing the 16 hour service learning requirement, students must submit: the Pediatric Respite Care Focus Sheet, Respite Journal and Journey paper by the end of the semester.

FIGURE 3.5   Student guidelines for respite clinical experience.

During the visit, the faculty reviews program guidelines with the parent(s) and the student and answers any questions. The family is provided with the student's name, phone number, and e-mail address and, if possible, the next respite visit is scheduled. The family is also given contact information for the faculty and encouraged to call with any concerns.

Student Assignments

After completing the 16-hour service learning requirement, students must submit a completed pediatric respite care focus sheet, respite journal, and journey paper. The focus sheet draws the student's attention to the care required by the child and the community services available to

SAINT MARY'S COLLEGE
DEPARTMENT OF NURSING
N326 CHILD HEALTH NURSING

PEDIATRIC RESPITE CARE FOCUS SHEET

1.   Briefly list the medical diagnosis(es) of this child.

2.   How do these diagnoses impact the:
      a)   child's physical growth/ developmental abilities?
      b)   child's psychosocial development?
      c)   family's dynamics?

3.   List all physician/specialists that provide care to the child (ex. Neurologist,
      gastroenterologist). Where is each physician's office/practice located (ex. South Bend,
      Indianapolis, Chicago)? How often does the child have appointments with each physician?

4.   What therapies does the child/family receive? (ex. OT, PT, speech therapy, therapeutic
      horseback riding, therapeutic swimming) How often does the child/family receive these
      therapies? (ex. Times/week) Are these therapies conducted in the home, school, or clinic?

5.   What types of alternate care/respite services does the family have in place (ex: home
      nursing, extended family, church/parish, friends)? How many hours/day &/or days/week (or
      month) does the family receive these services?

6.   Do the parents feel that they are provided adequate community support to care for their
      child/family? Explain

7.   What could be done to enhance the support provided to the child/family?

8.   Overall, how do you feel the family (parents, siblings, child) had adjusted to the child's
      physical/developmental disabilities?

FIGURE 3.6   Focus sheet assignment.

meet the child's needs (Figure 3.6). The journal is a tool that the student uses to keep track of each visit and to reflect on each individual respite experience. The journey paper requires that the student reflect on the meaning/benefit of the entire respite experience (Figure 3.7). Reflection provides a vital link between the service and the learning, and thus ensures that learning takes place (Butler, 2004; Eyler, 2002).

SAINT MARY'S COLLEGE
DEPARTMENT OF NURSING
N326 CHILD HEALTH NURSING

PEDIATRIC RESPITE CARE WRITTEN ASSIGNMENTS

1.   Focus sheet - to be submitted after completion of respite hours. (**20 points**)

2.   Respite Journal - the student should keep a journal of each of their respite visits. Each journal entry should include the following:
   a.   The date and time of respite visit
   b.   What you did while you were there
   c.   How the visit was a benefit to the members of the family (parent, child, siblings)
   d.   How you felt about the experience (what went well, what you would like to do differently next time)
   e.   What you plan to do (accomplish) during your next visit. (**20 points**)

3.   Journey Paper- After you have completed all of your respite hours, reflect on your overall respite experience. Examine your journal entries and reflect on the respite experience.
   a.   What expectations did you have prior to this experience?
   b.   Describe the most enjoyable aspect of your experience.
   c.   Describe the most frustrating aspect of your experience.
   d.   Describe the most surprising aspect of your experience.
   e.   What part of the experience was meaningful to you?
   f.   How did this experience influence your understanding of family?
   g.   How did this experience influence your understanding of chronic illness?
   h.   How did this experience influence your understanding of caring?
   i.   How did this experience influence your understanding of social responsibility?
   j.   What have you learned about yourself?
   k.   What have you learned about the needs of the community?

   Submit a paper that summarizes your reflections of the respite experience. Please include how this experience impacted you as an individual and how participating in the respite program will altered your nursing practice? (**100 points**)

FIGURE 3.7   Description of written assignments for respite experience.

Program Evaluation

The Time Out program is evaluated each semester by the parents, the students, and the course faculty. To date, the format used for the program evaluation has been qualitative in design. Open-ended questionnaires are used to solicit evaluative feedback from parents and students. Parents are asked to evaluate the student's effectiveness as a respite provider and also the overall program's ability to meet their needs. Students evaluate the learning experience and the parent's flexibility, responsibility, and need for respite care. Faculty evaluation of student learning and community service is accomplished by reviewing student assignments and student and parent evaluations. The journey paper serves as a synthesis of student learning, which is helpful for both student and faculty evaluation. Copies of evaluation forms are available by request.

Responses to the questionnaires and the journey papers are reviewed individually and collectively to identify the differing kinds of responses and to identify patterns in the data. The following themes emerged from analysis of the parent and student evaluations and the journey papers.

Parent Evaluation of the Time Out Program

Parents of children with special needs have so little community support that it is difficult to get them to provide candid feedback about the respite program. Parents fear that if they say something negative, they will be dropped from the respite program. The program coordinator has spent years trying to reassure parents that they will not lose respite services if they point out areas in which the program could be enhanced and that their comments are necessary if the program is going to better meet their future needs. Two examples of program changes that were directly related to parent input were described under program guidelines: the administration of feedings and medications by student respite providers. A third request for program enhancement was to increase the amount of time that each student is required to do. Initially, students were required to provide 14 hours of respite care; this was increased to 16 hours in 2001.

Parents are sent an evaluation form at the end of each semester. Evaluation return rates vary between 92–96%. Although it is not required that the families return the evaluations to continue in the program, it is stressed that parent feedback is critical for program refinement. Parent evaluations have been positive, reporting benefits for their child, themselves, and their family.

When asked, "How did the program benefit you?," one mother responded, "Time Out allowed me to exercise, do a little gardening, and do weekly grocery shopping (by myself). Having this time made me a better mother and a better wife." Another parent commented that the Time Out program "gave us time to eat out alone, get necessities done, and be better parents." Another parent wrote: "Time Out allowed us to take a breather and gather ourselves mentally, physically, and spiritually. It made us better and stronger parents both away from and with the children. Time Out brought back a quality of life that we have not had for many years."

Parents believed that the program benefited their other children as well. One mother wrote: "Both my husband and I could attend our 9-year-old's baseball game." Other parents responded: "It gave us an opportunity to do things with our other children that normally we can't do."

Parents also reported many benefits of the program for their child with special needs. The respite program "gave him an opportunity to interact with other people." Another commented, "He learned to respond to and build a relationship with a new person—a big deal for a child with autism."

One unexpected response made by several parents related to their satisfaction in assisting with the professional education of the student. "It has been an absolute pleasure watching her confidences and skills grow as she provided excellent, loving care to our daughter."

Student Evaluation of the Time Out Program

Like the program itself, student evaluation of the program has evolved over time. The initial evaluation simply assessed the student's level of exposure to children with special needs. Later evaluations attempted to rate student learning on a Likert-type scale. Both evaluations fell short of providing insight into the quality of learning associated with this service project. Anecdotally, faculty heard comments from students that indicated the respite experience had a profound effect on them, but early evaluations failed to capture this.

Journey Papers

It has been through the analysis of the journey papers that the faculty has been able to truly evaluate the impact of the program on student learning. Student comments such as: "This experience was an eye opener," and "I didn't realize how much we all take for granted" convey to the faculty that the students have met the learning objectives. While reviewing the journey papers submitted by the students, several common themes have been identified. One theme is that the respite experience has allowed students to gain insights into the daily lives of families with children with special needs. One student commented:

> K's mom has spent countless hours and energy trying to get the best care for K. Before this experience, I did not know how much time was involved in therapy. I didn't know so much money was spent on these programs when kids have such chronic conditions and I didn't know that a 14-month-old, who basically can't even move and has to keep his head elevated all the time, could be so much work.
>
> After each of my visits, I was exhausted. I can only imagine how much work his parents have to do.

Another theme was that students can see the hardships that caring for children with chronic illnesses can have on family members.

> It is obvious that both parents love Z a lot, but it is also apparent that caring for him is not easy. Their relationship is strained. There is also a lot of tension between Z and his younger brother. His younger brother told me 'It's no fun having a handicapped brother.'

After spending time with the family, students begin to see beyond the disability. One student remarked:

> Instead of focusing on the patient's illness, I am now able to look past that to see who the individual is inside.

The respite program also exposes students to the professional frustrations experienced by nurses in all areas of practice as they realize that, despite their good intentions, they cannot "fix it all." One student explained:

> After my initial meeting, I knew that this family needed more help than I could ever provide. I called my mom (a special education teacher) and one of the faculty who is a speech pathologist to get ideas on ways to help. I clearly had good intentions going in. Good intentions don't always mean good results. Even though I dreaded going back, I kept thinking of this mom and dad and how desperately they needed time away. Mom is there 24/7. She is getting burnt out. . . . On my last visit, the mom told me that they are trying to get E taken out of the home. When I first heard this I was shocked. My 16 hours was nothing compared to the time this family really needs. I wonder what else I could have done.

The respite experience enhances student confidence in their abilities. Many of the journey papers included descriptions by students of how much they learned from the experience and how their confidence improved. For example:

> The first day I just sat there like a deer in the headlights as Mrs. J introduced us individually to her six special needs foster children. On the second visit I came to appreciate their family and the dynamics it takes to keep things running "relatively" smoothly. Through the course of the semester, I learned not to take R's profanity and throwing things at me personally. I learned to stand taller when S and T were talking to me so loud that my eardrums felt like they were going to burst. I learned how to put two braces and two shoes on two kids as they were running out the door to play. This has been an amazing experience that every nursing major needs. It made me appreciate how orderly and easy my life is.

Faculty Lessons Learned

The Time Out program has been an eye opening experience for the nursing faculty. Prior to the development of the program, the pediatric nursing faculty's primary clinical experience was in the acute care setting. Transitioning from the hospital to the home brought a new understanding that has benefited faculty practice in and out of the hospital.

Developing program guidelines and enrolling families into the program was a growth experience that allowed the faculty to "look outside the box." The current program format requires the faculty to make introductory respite visits with each student. This results in a significant increase in faculty workload at the beginning of each semester. Workload is evened out later in the semester when the faculty have large blocks of time to use for other activities. Not being in clinical 12 or more hours every week frees up faculty time for scholarship and service.

The faculty member typically sees each family two to three times per year. These visits provide an opportunity for catchup on family news and the opportunity to witness how the child with special needs has grown and developed over the past few months. It is often difficult for family members to see progress on a day-to-day or week-to-week basis. Because the faculty member sees the child so infrequently, it is easy to notice the gains that the child has made over the past 4–6 months. Parents are grateful when the faculty can truthfully say, "Wow, look how he has grown," or "She is really sitting up much better than she did last fall when I was here."

An unexpected outcome of the program is the advocacy role that has evolved among faculty and parents. As the faculty gained experience working with families with children with special needs in the community, they became a valuable resource for the families. Parents quickly learned to use the expertise of the faculty to answer questions related to the care of their child, to find resources within the community, and to network with other families.

Summary

In the past 8 years, Saint Mary's College nursing students have provided more than 3,000 hours of respite services to 50 families (60 children with special needs) living in the community. The Time Out program has helped struggling families meet the day-to-day demands of their lives while enhancing the education of the students who are privileged to work with them. Participating in the respite program has allowed students to meet course objectives in a way that is meaningful. Students are able to see the application of theory and knowledge in a broader environment. By assisting families in the provision of care for their child students gain technical experiences as they witness the life and work of the family who must live with the need to be ever-caring and ever-vigilant of their child who is medically fragile. Participation in the respite program fosters the development of the more intangible aspects of nursing practice.

During one inpatient component of the pediatric rotation, the faculty overheard a staff nurse complaining that the parents of a patient with special needs hardly visited their child at all: "They are just in and out." The student caring for that child looked at the staff nurse and replied that this hospitalization is probably the only respite that this family has. The student demonstrated a better understanding of the issues faced by this family than the nurse who had been practicing for 10 years.

REFERENCES

American Association of Colleges of Nursing (AACN). (1999). *Nursing education's agenda for the 21st century* (position statement). Washington, DC: AACN.

Ashworth, M., & Baker, A. (2000). Time and space: Carer's views about respite care. *Health and Social Care in the Community, 8*(1), 50–56.

Bailey, P., Carpenter, D., & Harrington, P. (Eds.). (1999). *Integrating community service into nursing education: A guide to service learning.* New York: Springer Publishing.

Baum, L. (2004). Internet parent support groups for primary caregivers of a child with special health care needs. *Pediatric Nursing, 30*(5), 381–388.

Baumgardner, D., & Burtea, E. (1998). Quality-of-life in technology-dependent children receiving home care, and their families—A qualitative study. *Wisconsin Medical Journal, 97*(8), 51–55.

Brust, J., Leonard, B., & Sielaff, B. (1992). Maternal time and the care of disabled children. *Public Health Nursing, 9*(3), 177–184.

Butler, K. (2004). The use of critical reflection in baccalaureate nursing education. *Nursing Leadership Forum, 8*(4), 138–145.

Cernoch, J. (1992). Fact sheet number 11: Respite care for children who are medically fragile. Retrieved February 20, 2006, from www.archrespite.org/archfs11.html

Eyler, J. (2002). Reflecting on service: Helping nursing students get the most from service-learning. *Journal of Nursing Education, 41*, 453–456.

Folden, S., & Coffman, S. (1993). Respite care for families of children with disabilities. *Journal of Pediatric Health Care, 7*(3), 103–109.

Garth, R., Felicitti, D., & Sigmon, R. (2004). *Engaging communities and campuses— Building college and university capacity to engage with communities.* Washington, DC: Council of Independent Colleges.

Godshall, M. (2003). Caring for families of chronically ill kids. *RN, 66*(2), 30–35.

Harrigan, R., Ratliffe, C., Patrinos, M., & Tse, A. (2002). Medically fragile children: An integrative review of the literature and recommendations for future research. *Issues in Comprehensive Pediatric Nursing, 25*, 1–20.

Heaman, D. (1995). Perceived stressors and coping strategies of parents who have children with developmental disabilities: A comparison of mothers with fathers. *Journal of Pediatric Nursing, 10*, 311–319.

Higher Learning Commission (HLC). (2003). *Institutional accreditation: An overview.* Chicago: HLC.

Kendle, J., & Campanale, R. (2001). A pediatric learning experience: Respite care for families with children with special needs. *Nurse Educator, 26*(2), 95–98.

MacDonald, H., & Callery, P. (2004). Different meanings of respite: A study of parents, nurses and social workers caring for children with complex needs. *Child: Care, Health & Development, 30*(3), 279–288.

McManus, P., Fox, H., Newacheck, P., National Health Law Program, Perkins, J., Meldon, M., et al. (n.d.) Medicaid Waivers. Retrieved February 20, 2006, from http://www.familyvoices.org/Information/HCF.htm

Miller, S. (2002). Respite care for children who have complex healthcare needs. *Paediatric Nursing, 14*(5), 33–37.

Montagnino, B., & Mauricio, R. (2004). The child with a tracheostomy and gastrostomy: Parental stress and coping in the home—A pilot study. *Pediatric Nursing, 30*, 373–380.

Neufeld, S., Query, B., & Drummond, J. (2001). Respite care users who have children with chronic conditions: Are they getting a break? *Journal of Pediatric Nursing, 16*, 234–244.

Olsen, R., & Maslin-Prothero, P. (2001). Dilemmas in the provision of own-home respite support for evidence from an evaluation. *Journal of Advanced Nursing, 34*, 603–610.

Parish, S., Pomeranz, A., Hemp, R., Rizzolo, M., & Braddock, D. (2001). Family support for families of persons with developmental disabilities in the US: Status and trends. *Policy Research Brief: The College of Education and Human Development.* Minneapolis: University of Minnesota Press.

Parra, M. (2003, May). Nursing and respite care services for ventilator assisted children. *Caring,* 6–9.

Peterson, S., & Schaffer, M. (2001). Service-learning: Isn't that what nursing education has always been? *Journal of Nursing Education, 40*, 51–52.

Ray, L. (2002). Parenting and childhood chronicity: Making visible the invisible work. *Journal of Pediatric Nursing, 17*, 424–438.

Robinson, C., Jackson, P., & Townsley, R. (2001). Short breaks for families caring for a disabled child with complex health needs. *Child and Family Social Work, 6*, 67–75.

Rogers, M. (2001). Service learning resource allocation. *Nurse Educator, 26*, 244–247.

Seifer, S., & Vaughn, R. (2002). Partners in caring and community: Service-learning in nursing education. *Journal of Nursing Education, 41*, 437–439.

Sokol, M. (1995). Creating a community of caring for families with special needs. *Journal of Obstetric, Gynecologic, and Neonatal Nursing, 24*(1), 64–69.

Thurgate, C. (2005). Respite for children with complex health needs: Issues from the literature. *Paediatric Nursing, 17*(3), 14–18.

Thyen, U., Terres, N., Yazdgerdi, S., & Perrin, J. (1998). Impact of long-term care of children assisted by technology on maternal health. *Developmental and Behavioral Pediatrics, 19*, 273–282.

Treneman, M., Corkery, A., Dowdney, L., & Hammond, J. (1997). Respite-care needs— Met and unmet: Assessment of needs for children with disability. *Developmental Medicine & Child Neurology, 39*, 548–553.

Valkenier, B., Hayes, V., & McElheran, P. (2002). Mothers' perspectives of an in-home nursing respite service: Coping and control. *Canadian Journal of Nursing Research, 34*(1), 87–109.

Weingarten, C. (2003). Community classrooms: Service learning pairs nursing students, public schools. *Nursing Spectrum.* Retrieved February 3, 2006, from http://community.nursingspectrum.com/magazineArticles/article.cfm?AID= 9426

Withers, P., & Bennett, L. (2003). Myths and marital discord in a family with a child with profound physical and intellectual disabilities. *British Journal of Learning Disabilities, 31*, 91–95.

Chapter 4

Registered Nurses Mentoring Baccalaureate Nursing Students: Instrument Development and Preliminary Testing

Mary-Anne Andrusyszyn, Carroll L. Iwasiw, Dolly Goldenberg, Cathy Mawdsley, Barbara Sinclair, Charlene Beynon, Cathy Parsons, Kristen Lethbridge, and Richard Booth

Mentoring is a voluntary partnership in which an individual with knowledge and experience (*mentor*) acts as a role model, guide, and support, over an extended period of time, to facilitate a less experienced person's (*mentee's*) professional development (Committee on Science, Engineering, and Public Policy, 1997; Hayes, 1998), without formal evaluation. Mentoring is a form of leadership that can be enacted in all settings (Domino, 2005). Characterized by commitment, understanding, trust, and respect, mentoring promotes the mentee's current and future personal and professional interests and potential (Dorsey & Baker, 2004; Hayes, 1998; Jonson, 1998; Norman, 1997). The mentoring relationship results in reciprocal benefits through a spirit of sharing and learning (Clements, Mugavin, & Capitano, 2005; Hayes, 2005; Sword, Byrne, Drummond-Young, Harmer, & Rush, 2002).

Mentoring is viewed as a valuable component of nursing students' education (Dorsey & Baker, 2004; Nelson, Godfrey, & Purdy, 2004). Although there are several reports of nurses mentoring nursing students

---

This chapter was accepted on March 30, 2006.

in the United Kingdom (UK) and in North America, these are largely anecdotal (Dorsey & Baker, 2004; Jonson, 1998; Sword et al., 2002). Instruments to assess the characteristics and outcomes of mentoring in nursing education have not been described (Dorsey & Baker, 2004). This chapter describes the first phase of a 3-year research study about a formal mentoring program for first-year baccalaureate nursing (BScN) students (mentees) by RNs (mentors), funded by the Social Sciences and Humanities Research Council of Canada. In this phase, theoretically grounded questionnaires were developed to determine the nature and outcomes of the mentoring relationship for students and RNs. Background information is presented, followed by a summary of the pilot study. The development and pilot testing of the questionnaires are described, and the mentor pre-intervention questionnaire is included.

Background

Mentoring relationships are common in professional disciplines (Galicia, Klima, & Date, 1997; Hayes, 2005; Lee et al., 2006; Milner & Bossers, 2005; Ryan & Brewer, 1997). There is a wealth of literature describing the benefits of partnerships between experienced nurses and students. Dorsey and Baker's (2004) literature review on mentoring and retention of undergraduate nursing students "yielded over 90 citations, 51 of which were published between 1991 and 2003" (p. 261). Sixteen of these citations were research studies, conducted mostly in the UK, about mentoring nursing students. Unfortunately, the concepts of mentoring and preceptoring are used interchangeably in the nursing education literature, and the terms are often confused (Andrews & Wallis, 1999). The majority of these 16 citations addressed nurse–student relationships during clinical practice experiences throughout the educational program or in the final year (Cahill, 1996; Earnshaw, 1995; Lloyd Jones, Walters, & Ackehurst, 2001; Spouse, 1996). These partnerships were more closely aligned with preceptorships, that is, short-lived formal positions in which an experienced nurse helps a nursing student learn in the practice area as part of that student's educational program (Andrews & Chilton, 2000; Atkins & Williams, 1995; Gray & Smith, 2000; Milton, 2004; Morle, 1990; Pulsford, Boit, & Owen, 2002). Furthermore, formal appraisal is normally an important part of learning with a preceptor, whereas it is not part of a mentoring relationship. The roles of mentor and preceptor, therefore, should not be viewed as equivalent, nor are they compatible due to the fundamental dilemma of being model and judge simultaneously (Anforth, 1992).

Nursing education research that focused solely on mentorship (not preceptorship) of BScN students by RNs (without academic evaluation) was not found. Three expository articles describing mentorship programs by RNs with BScN students were located (Brown, 2004; Jonson, 1998; Sword et al., 2002). Brown described a program, offered through Bloomington Hospital in Indiana (in the United States), called "adopting a nursing student" (p. 242). Initiated as a recruitment/retention strategy, nurses volunteered to mentor senior nursing students. Brown reported that "the outcome of the student mentor program was more than statistics could express" (p. 243), with 89% of students choosing to work at that hospital post-graduation. Nurse mentors also benefited from the opportunity by "sharing their love and knowledge of the nursing profession" (p. 243).

Jonson (1998) reported on a mentoring program for students who were beginning the second year of their baccalaureate program. Volunteer nurse-mentors were assigned to students based on geographic location and remained paired until the student graduated, unless a change was requested by either partner. Mentor-mentee dyads were encouraged to meet and call each other regularly. Mentors provided whatever support, knowledge, advice, or expertise was requested by the mentee, ranging from suggesting topics for papers, to preparing for licensure examinations, and role-playing in preparation for a job interview. A 3-year post-program implementation evaluation revealed reciprocal benefits for mentors and mentees.

McMaster University School of Nursing in Canada initiated a mentoring program by nursing program alumni, who volunteered to be mentors for interested baccalaureate nursing students (Sword et al., 2002). Following a pilot study with 20 randomly matched pairs of mentors and students, this mentoring program expanded, and since its start in 1995, this program has grown to 146 participant pairs. Feedback obtained during annual social gatherings revealed the program was beneficial for both groups despite challenges associated with finding time to meet. Sword et al. confirmed that mentoring opportunities should be considered for nursing students "during their formative years" (p. 431).

In summary, research into the structure, process, and outcomes of formal mentoring programs for baccalaureate students by RNs, without the constraints associated with evaluation, is timely and indeed long overdue. The research study for which the instruments described in this chapter were developed takes up Sword et al.'s (2002) recommendation by focusing on the implementation and evaluation of formal mentoring of beginning BScN students by RNs.

Pilot Study

In 2003–2004, a qualitative pilot study was undertaken to explore the nature and merits of a formal mentoring relationship between RNs and first-year BScN students. The idea of establishing such a program for beginning nursing students was proposed by a clinical nurse specialist, Cathy Mawdsley (personal communication, November, 25, 2002), who had observed the benefits of extended formal mentorships between physicians and medical students. The specific goals of the pilot project were to determine the characteristics and outcomes of the mentoring relationship; rewards and challenges experienced by participants; and merits and feasibility of establishing formal mentoring relationships as part of the BScN program. Volunteers, 12 students and 12 RNs from one large quaternary hospital, were randomly selected and paired for the academic year.

Data pertinent to the four goals were collected through individual and focus group interviews. The results were very positive, and some mentor-mentee dyads were continuing their relationship 2 years later. The support from participants to pursue this initiative and make it available to a larger number of first year students led to the current 3-year funded study beginning in 2005. Phase 1, the first year, described herein, was devoted to the development of theory-based questionnaires that will be used to assess the mentoring relationships in the second and third phases of the study.

Instrument Development and Testing

Theoretical Frameworks

Researchers identified two important processes from the analysis of the pilot data, namely, empowerment and changed perspectives. First, students and nurses felt empowered and energized by their relationship, and described the activities and interactions that led to this outcome. Second, dyads related that their perspectives about a number of issues had changed or transformed. Nurses reflected and gained insights into their own as well as students' experiences and ideas; students saw the "real world" of nursing without the mediating influence of faculty. Congruent with the pilot data, *empowerment* and *perspective transformation* became the theoretical frameworks used to ground the study and the questionnaires. Our hypothesis for the larger study, therefore, was that the synergy associated with the mentoring relationship would lead to feelings of empowerment and transformed perspectives in students and nurses about nursing practice, the profession, and themselves.

Kanter's Theory of Structural Power in Organizations (1977; 1993) was chosen to assess empowerment in mentoring relationships. Although its origins are in organizational environments, Kanter's theory has recently been used to study empowerment structures in nursing education, and a good fit with educational practices has been demonstrated (Avolio, 1998; Ledwell, Andrusyszyn, & Iwasiw, in press; Sinclair, 2000; Siu, Laschinger, & Iwasiw, 2005). Kanter proposes that access to empowerment structures (information, resources, opportunities, and support) leads to self-efficacy, motivation, commitment, and job satisfaction. In relation to this study, it is anticipated that the mentoring relationship will provide students and nurses with access to these empowerment structures and that participants will be empowered as an outcome of the mentoring relationship.

Mezirow's (1990, 1991) Theory of Perspective Transformation seemed appropriate to determine changing outlooks during the mentoring relationship. According to Mezirow (1991),

> perspective transformation "begins when we encounter experiences... that fail to fit our expectations and consequently lack meaning for us, or we encounter an anomaly that cannot be given coherence either by learning within existing schemes or by learning new schemes" (p. 94).

Through perspective transformation, meaning structures are transformed as individuals engage in self-reflection, the central dynamic for learning (Daley, 1997), and new insights are gained about experiences. This theory has been used as a framework for nursing education studies with RN-BSN and graduate students (Callin, 1996; Cragg & Andrusyszyn, 2004; 2005). "Transformative learning is the mechanism by which [individuals] can adopt a broader, more inclusive view of nursing..." (Dingel-Stewart & LaCoste, 2004, p. 3).

Questionnaire Development Team

The research team is comprised of academics, clinicians of local agencies from which mentors will be recruited, and graduate students. The academics, experts in nursing education, and graduate students in the nursing education field of study developed the questionnaires. The clinicians, experienced in staff nurse mentoring programs and student clinical education, acted as external reviewers. They critiqued successive iterations of the questionnaires, offered ideas for items, and provided feedback about item clarity. Their expertise was beneficial and contributed to establishing content validity related to mentoring. Content validity related to the theoretical constructs was determined through comparisons with other instruments based on the two selected theories and examination by researchers on the team experienced in use of the theories. As is typical, content validity was determined by "interjudgemental consensus" (Maxim, 1999, p. 209).

Questionnaires Based on Theoretical Frameworks

The two theoretical frameworks provided the starting point for instrument development, and questionnaires were structured to match the major concepts of the theories. Items were generated from the theoretical frameworks, pilot data, literature about mentoring, and the knowledge and expertise of the research team. The original intent was to create four instruments based on Kanter's and Mezirow's theories: pre- and postmentorship questionnaires, with parallel versions for RNs and students. The prementorship questionnaires were designed to assess mentoring expectations, and the postmentorship questionnaires were intended to capture what had happened in the relationship. Figure 4.1, at the end of the chapter, displays the mentor pretest.

   Items on the pre- and postmentorship questionnaires were the same, although verb tense was changed to reflect relative time points. The RN and student questionnaires contained the same items, although they were written from the perspective of each respondent group. Instruments were developed through an iterative process, and each instrument underwent many changes with rewording and reordering of items before being finalized. A final step was to ensure that RN and student questionnaires and pre- and postquestionnaires corresponded exactly.

Additional Instruments

As progress was being made on the Kanter and Mezirow questionnaires, it became apparent that important ideas about the roles fulfilled by mentors did not fit these theoretical frameworks. Therefore, an additional questionnaire devoted to mentors' roles was constructed using Andrews and Chilton's (2000) description of mentor roles, and Brigham and Women's Hospital's (2004) online instrument *Measuring Mentoring Potential*, both adapted from Darling's (1984) work, and other ideas from the literature. Again, pre- and postmentorship questionnaires, with student and RN versions, were produced.

Questionnaires were also developed for control group participants. In addition to baseline demographic data, nurses were asked to respond to items based on their usual interactions with nursing students. Students were asked to respond to items on the basis of their expectations as they began and completed the first year of the nursing program.

Questionnaire Format

Concept labels were included in early versions of the questionnaires to help the researchers remain focused on theoretical elements. These were removed from the final version because of the potential influence on responses (Shaeffer & Presser, 2003).

The advantages of Web-based surveys led us to SurveyMonkey© as the secure site on which to mount the questionnaire. These advantages include ease of response for participants, as most have access to the Internet; reduced amount of missing data; lack of data entry errors; ability to download data for analysis (Polit & Beck, 2004; Strickland et al., 2003); and low cost and convenience for researchers, compared with printed questionnaire production, distribution, and return (Dillman, 2000). However, we recognized the need for printed questionnaires for respondents who preferred this format or had slow computers and made these available so as not to disenfranchise anyone.

Questionnaires were prepared, revised, and finalized in a word processing program. Attention was paid to layout, item clarity, bias, logical

sequencing, and cognitive burden so that the items would be meaningful and reduce nonresponse (Dillman, 2000; Loiselle, Profetto-McGrath,
Polit, & Tantato-Beck, 2007). All the items were entered into the Web-
based software program using a combination of scrolling and screen-by-
screen construction methods (Dillman, 2000). This would allow respondents to complete conceptually organized segments of the questionnaire
and proceed to subsequent sections by clicking on "next" without having
to scroll through the whole questionnaire.

Some demographic items with multiple response categories did not
translate easily to the online format and had to be adjusted. The differences between the paper-based visual layout and computer-screen design features (Dillman, 2000) meant dividing the question into parts so
each part could be addressed separately. For example, the following demographic question had to be split into three parts (month/day/letters):

> Please enter the month and day of your birthday and the first two letters of
> your mother's maiden name (e.g., April 4 Adams (04 04 AD; November 12
> Smith ⇒ 11 12 SM
>
> _____   _____   _____
> Month   Day   First 2 letters of mother's maiden name

Online formatting also included attention to color choice to dif-
ferentiate items and make the questionnaires visually appealing. Colors
with "cultural" meaning were avoided (e.g., green for go; red for stop)
(Dillman, 2000). The questionnaires also were tested on different Web
browsers, and with different screen sizes to evaluate text size, align-
ment, and overall visual display so differences across respondents could
be minimized (Dillman).

Each set of questionnaires (e.g., all pre-mentorship and demographic questionnaires) for students and for RNs were mounted seam-
lessly as one continuous instrument. It was felt that asking participants to
respond to one questionnaire would be simpler than responding to several. This would also reduce the response time, because a reorientation to
each part of the questionnaire was not necessary. The online questionnaire was designed with scroll functions within conceptually parallel
sections of the questionnaire. As well, it used a screen-by-screen approach between the sections with navigational guides (Dillman, 2000).

Response Format. The response format is an opinion scale to which
participants indicate their extent of agreement with statements about the

mentoring relationship. Because the number of categories is unrelated to overall reliability and validity (Maxim, 1999), an early decision was that seven gradations of agreement were excessive and that either four or five options were sufficient. Considerable attention was given to inclusion or exclusion of a midpoint on the opinion scale, with full discussion of the advantages and disadvantages of each. Finally, the neutral position was included to improve response variance. As well, we were persuaded by the argument that lack of a midpoint can lead participants to become annoyed and decide not to complete the questionnaire. The two ends of the response scale were anchored with descriptors.

Because the questionnaires would be distributed electronically, and the program only allows the respondent to leave blank or change, but not delete, a response once entered, the university's research ethics board directed that we include a sixth option. *No response* was added for participants who preferred not to respond to a particular item. The forced-choice feature, an option in SurveyMonkey©, requiring a response to an item before being allowed to proceed to the next one, was not used (Dillman, 2000).

Instrument Testing

Sixteen 1st and 3rd-year BScN students and 12 RNs pilot-tested the Internet-based questionnaire. Third-year students were specifically chosen, as we hoped that some of the students who participated in the pilot study might respond to the questionnaires. It was not expected that participants had experienced a mentoring relationship, and we asked that they provide feedback based on their opinion of the clarity and meaning of items; familiarity with the terminology used; and whether items were understandable, intrusive, loaded, or offensive. They were also asked to comment on access to the survey Web site and ease of use of the software. Due to the nature of the pilot study, internal consistency was not assessed.

In addition, pilot participants provided qualitative information online about the questions, data collection protocol, and use of the Internet format. They reported that the meaning of items was clear, and the procedures were easy to follow. We learned that the format of the questionnaire was altered by some Internet browsers. Specifically, bullets placed in front of each item were corrupted into various symbols and, consequently, these were removed from the electronic version.

Conclusion

In this chapter, the development of questionnaires for a 3-year funded study about mentoring of first-year BScN students by RNs was described. Psychometric testing will be undertaken when data are collected through 2006–2008. Testing will be conducted separately for Internet and print versions of the questionnaires because differences can exist (Strickland et al., 2003). Although refinements may be necessary as testing proceeds, these instruments contribute to nursing education scholarship by providing a theoretically based means to assess formal RN-BScN student mentoring.

REFERENCES

Andrew, M., & Wallis, M. (1999). Mentorship in nursing: A literature review. *Journal of Advanced Nursing, 29*, 201–207.

Andrews, M., & Chilton, F. (2000). Student and mentor perceptions of mentoring effectiveness. *Nurse Education Today, 20*, 555–562.

Anforth, P. (1992). Mentors, not assessors. *Nurse Education Today, 12*, 299–302.

Atkins, S., & Williams, A. (1995). Registered nurses' experiences of mentoring undergraduate nursing students. *Journal of Advanced Nursing, 21*, 1006–1015.

Avolio, J. (1998). *Perceptions of empowering teaching behaviours and nursing students' self efficacy for professional nursing practice.* Unpublished master's thesis, The University of Western Ontario, London, Ontario, Canada.

Brigham and Women's Hospital. (2004). Measuring mentoring potential: Women's Hospital Miriam Walsh Diversity Mentor Award 2004. Retrieved March 25, 2006, from http://www.brighamandwomens.org/cne/walsh2004eval.doc

Brown, T. (2004). Adopting a nursing student. *Journal for Nursing Staff Development, 20*, 242–243.

Cahill, H. (1996). A qualitative analysis of student nurses' experiences of mentorship. *Journal of Advanced Nursing, 24*, 791–799.

Callin, M. (1996). From RN to BSN: Seeing familiar situations in different ways. *The Journal of Continuing Education in Nursing, 27*, 28–33.

Clements, P. T., Mugavin, M., & Capitano, C. (2005). Mentorship in forensic research: Promoting the next generation of forensic nurse scientists. *Journal of Forensic Nursing, 1*, 129–132.

Committee on Science, Engineering, and Public Policy. (1997). Adviser, teacher, role model, friend: On being a mentor to students in science and engineering. National Academy Press: Washington, DC. Retrieved March 19, 2006, from http://www.nap.edu/readingroom/books/mentor/index.html

Cragg, C. E. (Betty), & Andrusyszyn, M. A. (2004). Outcomes of master's education in nursing. *International Journal of Nursing Education Scholarship, 1*(1), 1–20, Article 18. Retrieved March 25, 2006, from http://www.bepress.com/ijnes/vol1/iss1/art18

Cragg, C. E. (Betty), & Andrusyszyn, M. A. (2005). The process of master's education in nursing: Evolution or revolution? *International Journal of Nursing Education Scholarship, 2*(1), 1–15, Article 21. Retrieved March 25, 2006, from http://www.bepress.com/ijnes/vol2/iss1/art21

Daley, J. (1997). Transformative learning: Theory to practice links. Retrieved March 25, 2006, from http://www.anrecs.msu.edu/research/daley.htm

Darling, L. A. (1984). What do nurses want in a mentor? *Journal of Nursing Administration (JONA), 14*(10), 42–44.

Dillman, D. A. (2000). *Mail and Internet surveys: The tailored design method* (2nd ed.). New York: John Wiley & Sons, Inc.

Dingel-Stewart, S., & LaCoste, J. (2004). Light at the end of the tunnel: A vision for an empowered nursing profession across the continuum of care. *Nursing Administration Quarterly, 28,* 212–216.

Domino, E. (2005). Nurses are what nurses do-Are you where you want to be? *Association of Operating Room Nurses Journals, 81,* 187–201.

Dorsey, L., & Baker, C. M. (2004). Mentoring undergraduate nursing students. *Nurse Educator, 29,* 260–265.

Earnshaw, G. J. (1995). Mentorship: The students' views. *Nurse Education Today. 15,* 274–279.

Galicia, A. R., Klima, R. R., & Date, E. S. (1997). Mentorship in physical medicine and rehabilitation residencies. *American Journal of Physical Medicine and Rehabilitation, 76,* 268–275.

Gray, M. A., & Smith, L. N. (2000). The qualities of an effective mentor from the student nurse's perspective: Findings from a longitudinal qualitative study. *Journal of Advanced Nursing, 32,* 1542–1549.

Hayes, E. F. (1998). Mentoring and nurse practitioner student self-efficacy. *Western Journal of Nursing Research, 20,* 521–535.

Hayes, E. F. (2005). Approaches to mentoring: How to mentor and be mentored. *Journal of the American Academy of Nurse Practitioners, 17,* 442–445.

Kanter, R. M. (1977). *Men and women of the corporation.* New York: Basic Books.

Kanter, R. M. (1993). *Men and women of the corporation* (2nd ed.). New York: Basic Books.

Jonson, K. (1998). Learning the ropes through mentoring. *The Canadian Nurse, 94*(2) 27–30.

Ledwell, E., Andrusyszyn, M. A., & Iwasiw, C. (in press). Nursing students' empowerment in distance education: Testing Kanter's theory. *Journal of Distance Education.*

Lee, S.-H., Theoharis, R., Fitzpatrick, M., Kim, K.-H., Nix-Williams, T., Griswold, D. E., & Wealther-Thomas, C. (2006). Create effective mentoring relationships: Strategies for mentor and mentee success. *Intervention in School and Clinic, 41,* 233–240.

Lloyd Jones, M., Walters, S., & Akehurst, R. (2001). The implications of contact with the mentor for pre-registration nursing and midwifery students. *Journal of Advanced Nursing, 35*(2), 51–60.

Loiselle, C. G., Profetto-McGrath, J., Polit, D. F., & Tantato-Beck, C. (2007). *Polit and Beck: Canadian essentials of nursing research* (2nd ed.). Philadelphia: Lippincott Williams & Wilkins.

Maxim, P. S. (1999). Measurement theory. In *Quantitative research methods in the social sciences* (pp. 201–232). New York: Oxford University Press.

Mezirow, J. (1990). *Fostering critical reflection in adulthood: A guide to transformative and emancipatory learning.* San Francisco: Jossey-Bass, Inc.

Mezirow, J. (1991). *Transformative dimensions of adult learning.* San Francisco: Jossey-Bass, Inc.

Milner, T., & Bossers, A. (2005). Evaluation of an occupational therapy mentorship program. *The Canadian Journal of Occupational Therapy, 72*, 205–211.

Milton, C. (2004). The ethics of personal integrity in leadership and mentorship: A nursing theoretical perspective. *Nursing Science Quarterly, 17*, 116–120.

Morle, K. M. (1990). Mentorship—Is it a case of the emperor's new clothes, or a rose by any other name? *Nurse Education Today, 10*(1), 66–69.

Nelson, D., Godfrey, L., & Purdy, J. (2004). Using a mentorship program to recruit and retain student nurses. *Journal of Nursing Administration (JONA), 34*, 551–553.

Norman, E. M. (1997). Boosting your career with a mentor. *Orthopaedic Nursing, 16*(4), 13–16.

Polit, D. F., & Beck C.T. (2004). *Nursing research: Principles and methods* (7th ed.). Philadelphia: Lippincott Williams & Wilkins.

Pulsford, D., Boit, K., & Owen, S. (2002). Are mentors ready to make a difference? A survey of mentors' attitudes towards nurse education. *Nurse Education Today, 22*, 439–446.

Ryan, D., & Brewer, K. (1997). Mentorship and professional role development in undergraduate nursing education. *Nurse Educator, 22*(6), 22–26.

Shaeffer, N. C., & Presser, S. (2003). The science of asking questions. *American Review of Sociology, 29*, 65–88.

Sinclair, B. (2000). *An explanatory study of Kanter's theory: Empowerment in nursing education.* Unpublished master's thesis, The University of Western Ontario, London, Ontario, Canada.

Siu, H. M., Laschinger, H. K. S., & Vingilis, E. (2005). Empowerment in the learning environment: A comparative study between PBL and a conventional learning environment. *Journal of Nursing Education, 44*, 459–469.

Spouse, J. (1996). The effective mentor: A model for student-centered learning. *Nursing Times, 92*(13), 32–35.

Strickland, O. L., Moloney, M. F., Dietrich, A. S., Myerburg, S., Cotsonis, G., & Johnson, R. (2003). Measurement issues related to data collection on the World Wide Web. *Advances in Nursing Science, 26*, 246–256.

Sword, W., Byrne, C., Drummond-Young, M., Harmer, M., & Rush, J. (2002). Nursing alumni as student mentors: Nurturing professional growth. *Nurse Education Today, 22*, 407–432.

MENTORING OF BACCALAUREATE NURSING STUDENTS
BY REGISTERED NURSES

(MENTOR)

Thank you for agreeing to complete the first questionnaire about mentoring of baccalaureate students by registered nurses. As you respond to the questions, consider your participation in a mentoring relationship with a nursing student for the upcoming academic year. The purpose of the mentoring relationship is to help the student learn about the real world of nursing, and to discuss any other matters that might arise.

The questionnaire will take you approximately 10-15 minutes to complete.

Please send your responses to:

Dr. Mary-Anne Andrusyszyn
Associate Professor
School of Nursing
University of Western Ontario
London, ON N6A 5C1
maandrus@uwo.ca

FIGURE 4.1   Mentor pre-test.

MENTOR PRE-TEST ©

Please fill in your response to each of the items below:

A. Please enter the month and day of your birthday and the first two letters of your mother's maiden name (e.g., April 4 Adams → 04 04 AD; November 12 Smith → 11 12 SM)

_____   _____   _____

Month   Day   First 2 letters of mother's maiden name

Please choose the extent to which you agree with the following statements, where **1** = **strongly disagree** and **5** = **strongly agree**. If you prefer **not to respond** to any item, choose **N/R.**

1. THROUGH MY USUAL INTERACTIONS WITH NURSING STUDENTS, I BELIEVE THAT I HAVE ACCESS TO:	Strongly Disagree			Strongly Agree		N/R
• opportunities for professional development	1	2	3	4	5	N/R
• information that will contribute to my professional development	1	2	3	4	5	N/R
• resources that will contribute to my professional development	1	2	3	4	5	N/R
• support that will contribute to my professional development	1	2	3	4	5	N/R
2. IN MY USUAL INTERACTIONS WITH NURSING STUDENTS, I	Strongly Disagree			Strongly Agree		N/R
• build confidence in the role of nursing student	1	2	3	4	5	N/R
• engage in self-examination	1	2	3	4	5	N/R
• critically assess personal assumptions	1	2	3	4	5	N/R
• recognize that others have had similar difficulties	1	2	3	4	5	N/R
• know that I am there for support	1	2	3	4	5	N/R
• explore their role as a nursing student	1	2	3	4	5	N/R
• deal with dilemmas encountered in the nursing program	1	2	3	4	5	N/R

• discuss actions as a nursing student	1	2	3	4	5	N/R
• plan a course of action to be successful in nursing	1	2	3	4	5	N/R
• acquire competencies to be successful in nursing	1	2	3	4	5	N/R
• try new activities	1	2	3	4	5	N/R
• assess outcomes of new activities	1	2	3	4	5	N/R
• build competence in the role of nursing student	1	2	3	4	5	N/R
• integrate a new perspective on professional life	1	2	3	4	5	N/R
3. BY BEING A MENTOR TO A NURSING STUDENT, I BELIEVE THAT:	Strongly Disagree			Strongly Agree		N/R
• my expertise as a registered nurse will be more visible within my employment setting.	1	2	3	4	5	N/R
• I will be better known within my employment setting.	1	2	3	4	5	N/R
4. BY BEING A MENTOR TO A NURSING STUDENT, I BELIEVE THAT I WILL MAKE MORE CONNECTIONS WITH:	Strongly Disagree			Strongly Agree		N/R
• my colleagues	1	2	3	4	5	N/R
• baccalaureate nursing students	1	2	3	4	5	N/R
• the baccalaureate nursing program	1	2	3	4	5	N/R
5. BY BEING A MENTOR TO A NURSING STUDENT, I BELIEVE THAT IT WILL GIVE ME ACCESS TO:	Strongly Disagree			Strongly Agree		N/R
• opportunities for professional development	1	2	3	4	5	N/R
• information that will contribute to my professional development	1	2	3	4	5	N/R
• resources that will contribute to my professional development	1	2	3	4	5	N/R

• support that will contribute to my professional development	1	2	3	4	5	N/R
6. BY BEING A MENTOR TO A NURSING STUDENT, I BELIEVE THAT I WILL:	Strongly Disagree				Strongly Agree	N/R
• feel more motivated in my nursing role	1	2	3	4	5	N/R
• see greater value in the nursing profession	1	2	3	4	5	N/R
• feel more confident in my nursing role	1	2	3	4	5	N/R
• feel more independent in my nursing role	1	2	3	4	5	N/R
• feel more satisfied in my nursing role	1	2	3	4	5	N/R
• feel renewed commitment to the nursing profession	1	2	3	4	5	N/R
• feel more enthusiastic in my nursing role	1	2	3	4	5	N/R
• feel respected for being a mentor	1	2	3	4	5	N/R
• feel proud about facilitating a nursing student's professional development	1	2	3	4	5	N/R
• develop new understandings about nursing students' perspectives	1	2	3	4	5	N/R
• gain new understandings about how students can contribute to my learning	1	2	3	4	5	N/R
• gain new understandings about mentoring	1	2	3	4	5	N/R
7. BY BEING A MENTOR TO A NURSING STUDENT, I BELIEVE THAT I WILL:	Strongly Disagree				Strongly Agree	N/R
• have greater influence on the outcomes of my nursing work	1	2	3	4	5	N/R
• be more effective in my nursing role	1	2	3	4	5	N/R
• be better able to seek feedback about my nursing work	1	2	3	4	5	N/R
• acquire information I need	1	2	3	4	5	N/R
• be able to contribute more meaningfully to interdisciplinary practice	1	2	3	4	5	N/R

• be better able to provide feedback to students	1	2	3	4	5	N/R
• be better able to provide feedback to novice nurses	1	2	3	4	5	N/R
• involve nursing students in my work more than in the past	1	2	3	4	5	N/R
• help novice nurses more than in the past	1	2	3	4	5	N/R
• seek other opportunities to support nursing students	1	2	3	4	5	N/R
• promote a positive learning environment for students	1	2	3	4	5	N/R
• promote a positive work environment for novice nurses	1	2	3	4	5	N/R
• positively influence nurse retention	1	2	3	4	5	N/R

You have completed half of the questionnaire so far.

Please choose the extent to which you agree with the following statements, where **1 = strongly disagree** and **5 = strongly agree.** If you prefer **NOT TO RESPOND** to any item, choose **N/R.**

8. IN MY RELATIONSHIP WITH MY MENTEE, I EXPECT TO OFFER ADVICE ABOUT:	Strongly Disagree			Strongly Agree		N/R
• courses (e.g., assignments, electives)	1	2	3	4	5	N/R
• nursing practice	1	2	3	4	5	N/R
• the nursing profession	1	2	3	4	5	N/R
• personal matters (e.g., relationships)	1	2	3	4	5	N/R
• non-nursing matters (e.g., housing)	1	2	3	4	5	N/R
9. IN MY RELATIONSHIP WITH MY MENTEE, I EXPECT TO HELP MY MENTEE UNDERSTAND:	Strongly Disagree			Strongly Agree		N/R
• courses (e.g., assignments, electives)	1	2	3	4	5	N/R
• nursing practice	1	2	3	4	5	N/R
• the nursing profession	1	2	3	4	5	N/R
• personal matters (e.g., relationships)	1	2	3	4	5	N/R
• non-nursing matters (e.g., housing)	1	2	3	4	5	N/R

• what it takes to be successful in nursing	1	2	3	4	5	N/R
10. IN MY RELATIONSHIP WITH MY MENTEE, I EXPECT THE MENTEE TO:	Strongly Disagree			Strongly Agree		N/R
• sometimes question what I am saying	1	2	3	4	5	N/R
• consider ideas additional to those discussed	1	2	3	4	5	N/R
• reflect on ideas to see how he/she could improve	1	2	3	4	5	N/R
• reappraise the experience with me and learn from it	1	2	3	4	5	N/R

Please choose the extent to which you agree with the following statements, where **1 = strongly disagree** and **5 = strongly agree.** If you prefer **NOT TO RESPOND** to any item, choose **N/R.**

11. AS A RESULT OF THIS EXPERIENCE, I EXPECT MY MENTEE TO:	Strongly Disagree			Strongly Agree		N/R
• challenge his/her own firmly held ideas	1	2	3	4	5	N/R
• alter usual ways of thinking and approaching situations	1	2	3	4	5	N/R
• re-evaluate what was previously believed to be right	1	2	3	4	5	N/R
• change views of self as a person	1	2	3	4	5	N/R
• change views of self as a professional	1	2	3	4	5	N/R
12. MY RELATIONSHIP WITH MY MENTEE WILL HELP HIM/HER TO:	Strongly Disagree			Strongly Agree		N/R
• build confidence in the role of nursing student	1	2	3	4	5	N/R
• engage in self-examination	1	2	3	4	5	N/R
• critically assess personal assumptions	1	2	3	4	5	N/R
• recognize that others have had similar difficulties	1	2	3	4	5	N/R
• know that I am there for support	1	2	3	4	5	N/R
• explore their role as a nursing student	1	2	3	4	5	N/R

• deal with dilemmas encountered in the nursing program	1	2	3	4	5	N/R
• discuss actions as a nursing student	1	2	3	4	5	N/R
• plan a course of action to be successful in nursing	1	2	3	4	5	N/R
• acquire competencies to be successful in nursing	1	2	3	4	5	N/R
• try new activities	1	2	3	4	5	N/R
• assess outcomes of new activities	1	2	3	4	5	N/R
• build competence in the role of nursing student	1	2	3	4	5	N/R
• integrate a new perspective on professional life	1	2	3	4	5	N/R

Please choose the extent to which you agree that the following activities are part of your role as mentor, where **1 = strongly disagree** and **5 = strongly agree.** If you prefer **NOT TO RESPOND** to any item, choose **N/R.**

13. ACTIVITIES AS MENTOR	Strongly Disagree			Strongly Agree		N/R
• role modelling	1	2	3	4	5	N/R
• coaching	1	2	3	4	5	N/R
• providing intellectual stimulation	1	2	3	4	5	N/R
• educating	1	2	3	4	5	N/R
• counselling	1	2	3	4	5	N/R
• being an advocate	1	2	3	4	5	N/R
• being a friend	1	2	3	4	5	N/R
• providing advice about the nursing profession	1	2	3	4	5	N/R
• providing advice about nursing practice	1	2	3	4	5	N/R
• being a sounding board	1	2	3	4	5	N/R
• challenging ideas	1	2	3	4	5	N/R
• being a visionary	1	2	3	4	5	N/R
• providing support and encouragement	1	2	3	4	5	N/R

Please choose the extent to which you agree with the following statement, where **1 = strongly disagree** and **5 = strongly agree.** If you prefer **NOT TO RESPOND**, choose **N/R.**

14. OVERALL, I EXPECT THE MENTORING EXPERIENCE TO BE WORTHWHILE	1	2	3	4	5	N/R

The last group of questions focus on demographic information. You are almost done!

DEMOGRAPHICS

Please fill in your response to each of the items below:

1. Age (on last birthday).
    _____

2. Gender
    Male _____
    Female_____

3. Total years and months of experience in nursing.
    Years _____ and Months _____

4. Current position(s) and employment status (please check all that apply).

	Full Time	Part-time	Casual
Staff Nurse			
CNS/NP			
Educator			
Nurse Manager			
Professional Practice Leader			

5. If your position is not listed above in question 4, please specify your current position and employment status (e.g., consultant, part-time).
    _____

6. Average number of hours worked per week in nursing.
    _____

7. Length of time in current position. (If you have more than one position, respond to this for the position in which you spend the most time).
    Years _____ and Months _____

8. Previous Education:
Nursing Diploma _____
BScN _____
MScN _____
PhD _____
Other (please specify) _____

9. Are you *currently* enrolled in formal education? If yes, please select the appropriate response(s) below:
BScN _____
MScN _____
PhD _____
Certificate _____
Regular In-services _____
Nursing Specialty Courses _____
Other (please specify) -
_____

10. Have you ever had a preceptor? (*Preceptor*: a formal position in which an experienced individual helps a student learn in the practice area as part of the student's educational program.)
Yes _____
No _____

11. If you answered "Yes" to question 11, please describe your involvement.

12. Have you ever been a preceptor?
Yes _____
No _____

13. If you answered "Yes" to question 12, please describe your involvement.

14. Have you ever had a mentor? (*Mentor*: an individual with knowledge and experience who acts as a role model, guide, and support, over an extended period of time, to facilitate another individual's development as a successful professional.)
Yes _____
No _____

15. If you answered "Yes" to question 15, please describe your involvement.

16. Have you ever been a mentor?
    Yes   ____
    No   ____

17. If you answered "Yes" to question 17, please describe your involvement.

Thank you for completing this questionnaire.

Source: Reprinted by permission of Andrusyszyn, M.A., Iwasiw, C., Goldenberg, D., Mawdsley, C., Sinclair, B., Beynon, C., Parsons, C., Lethbridge, K., & Booth, R., April 4, 2006.

Part II

Challenges Faced by Nurse Educators

Chapter 5

Managing Difficult Student Situations: Lessons Learned

Susan Luparell

Although the National League for Nursing (2002) has called for change in how nursing faculty are prepared, the vast majority of current faculty transitioned into nursing education with little instruction on how to be educators. Those with no formal preparation in curriculum development and teaching methods typically did not receive extensive guidance on how to deal with the various challenging student situations that may arise, including how to facilitate learning for students with physical or learning disabilities, mental health issues, and multiple personal and professional role responsibilities.

Truth be told, I was more than a little surprised to find the student challenges that awaited me in the academic world. I had expected students to show up on time; complete their assignments conscientiously; and treat me, my colleagues, and each other in a professional and respectful manner. Thankfully, the majority of students meet this description. However, most of us occasionally encounter students who fall outside these parameters, and we find ourselves faced with the dilemma of how to best handle the various challenges presented. Additionally, some aspects of faculty work, such as administering a failing grade, are by their nature unpleasant and challenging, even in the best of circumstances.

As a still novice educator, I became especially interested in the challenges nurse educators face in their interactions with students when

This chapter was accepted on March 30, 2006.

I encountered a student who, in addition to her inability to achieve course objectives, was rude, indignant, and inappropriate. I have since learned that many instructors encounter students with similar dispositions. A national survey of nursing faculty confirmed that educators are confronted with problematic student behavior in astonishingly high numbers (Lashley & deMeneses, 2001). In addition to being yelled at both in the classroom (52.8%) and in the clinical setting (42.8%), almost one in four faculty respondents reported having experienced objectionable physical contact from a student. Strategies to prevent and address this type of incivility have been suggested and include delineating behavioral expectations, developing immediacy skills, and honing feedback skills (Luparell, 2005). Unfortunately, it appears that some of us are so surprised by inappropriate student behaviors that we are left unable to muster an effective response (Luparell, 2004).

Over the years, I have had a chance to reflect on the challenging student situations I have faced, particularly those associated with delivering constructive feedback and dealing with rude, unprofessional, or inappropriate behavior. As is often the case, the best lessons present themselves in the aftermath of failure, loss, or defeat. The purpose of this chapter is to share some of the mistakes I have made, as well as the lessons learned, in dealing with difficult or challenging student situations as a nurse educator.

Lesson 1: Concerns Should Not Be Ignored

As a new instructor, there were times I had concerns about student behavior that needed to be addressed, yet I hesitated to do so. For example, I mistakenly thought that placing demands on classroom behavior would be oppressive and stifling to student learning. I wanted the classroom to be a safe environment that facilitated learning; I wanted students to think that my classes were engaging and fun. Not that I invited classroom chaos, but I did want the classroom to be informal and creative. I am one who does not mind a few side comments in class, as I tend to think that some students learn better given the chance to quietly and quickly reiterate points by sharing an experience with a neighbor. However, there were times the side chatter was clearly not related to class or a comment was made that was not appropriate. Not wanting to appear overbearing, I tended to ignore these "minor" infractions, considering them isolated incidents that would likely resolve on their own. And sometimes they did. More often than not, however, the isolated incidents became recurrent. By not addressing the behavior, I had unwittingly sanctioned it.

There can be compounding problems when concerns you have about a student's behavior are not addressed early. First, the issue can grow bigger. It is easier to address a small issue early than to address a malignant issue later. A pair of students talking too much in class can quickly become a room full of students talking too much. The second or third time a student arrives late to the clinical unit can become a smudge on a program's reputation. I have found—particularly with concerns about a student's clinical performance—that the longer I wait to address a concern, the more difficult it is to address. A student may be confused or even resentful that a behavior that was not a problem has suddenly become one. Students need adequate time to make adjustments, and when there is delay in notifying them of a problem with performance, there may be a valid argument that insufficient notice was given to allow for correction of the problem. Thus, a little effort up front may save a lot of effort later.

Some behaviors demand even more pressing intervention. As tempting as it is to hope a problem behavior will go away on its own, we need to bear in mind that the Code of Ethics for Nurses (American Nurses Association, 2001) calls for respectful relationships with professional colleagues as well as patients. Thus, educators are ethically bound to address disrespectful behavior by students.

Lesson 2: The Instructor Is Responsible for the Learning Environment

This lesson is a direct extension of the previous lesson. It is important to note that students are keen observers of classroom dynamics. They observe how instructors handle various situations and form conclusions based on their responses. In particular, they may become disengaged, angry, or resentful if the faculty does not address a situation that should be addressed.

As a more seasoned instructor, I set the stage for classroom expectations on the first day of class. I tell the students that, although I do not mind a small amount of talking in class to facilitate learning, I am responsible for maintaining an environment that is conducive to every-one's learning. I let the students know that I will, therefore, be observant of the environment and may speak privately with individuals if behavior (e.g., talking in class or arriving late) seems to be affecting the learning of others.

How can an instructor determine if the environment is negatively affecting student learning? In addition to observation, one strategy is to ask the students. Some readers may be familiar with the 1-minute exercise, in which students are given 1 minute at the end of the class period to identify the salient points from that class and to ask for clarification about anything that remains unclear. This exercise can be adapted to help the instructor gain feedback about the classroom environment. Try handing out note cards at intervals during the semester and ask students to comment specifically on the classroom environment. Depending on your comfort level, you can ask specific questions about the learning environment or you can leave it open-ended. Students can identify undue distractions and make suggestions for attending to the problem.

Lesson 3: Make Trust the Essential Theme in Giving Feedback

Most students are unaccustomed to the type of feedback required to develop skilled professionals. As a novice, I began to notice that students appeared to regard faculty feedback, particularly constructive or negative feedback, as arbitrary. Additionally, the belief that students are "weeded out" of nursing programs appeared to be pervasive. Thus, it dawned on me that students had little understanding of the process of nursing education.

In my initial meeting with students, I try to establish trust as the essential theme in giving feedback. To ask for blind trust can be a tall order, especially if there is no prior relationship between instructor and students. Nonetheless, I do spend time on the first day of class explaining what drives my approach to giving feedback. I start by asking the class to raise their hands if they hope to become a mediocre nurse. I have yet to see a hand raised in response. I then ask who hopes to become a skilled and competent nurse. Usually, all hands go up. At this point, I share my philosophy on trust and the important role of honest feedback in my class. I trust that students are there because they want to achieve their goals. Thus, I trust that they want to hear feedback from me that will move them in that direction. I ask that they subsequently trust that the primary reason I give feedback is because I am committed to helping them achieve their goals. I remind the students of the role of trust each time I need to share constructive feedback with them. Since I began making the role of trust in giving and receiving feedback explicit from the outset, I cannot recall any difficulty administering feedback nor with students reacting badly to it.

Lesson 4: Say What You Mean and Mean What You Say

I used to marvel at how my mentor could look and sound so matter of fact when delivering constructive feedback to students, especially the kind associated with an unsatisfactory clinical day or a failing class grade. When it came my time to deliver this type of constructive feedback, my voice would quiver and my hands would tremble. It was both physically and emotionally uncomfortable for me, and I know it was psychologically uncomfortable for the student involved. The intense level of discomfort mistakenly led me to conclude that the feedback process itself was somehow uncaring. In a misguided attempt to minimize the discomfort and demonstrate caring, I usually went overboard in trying to soften the blow. Generally, I did so by softening the words. The problem with soft words is that often they do not convey the hard truth. Also, I relied heavily on the sandwich technique (what the student does well, what needs to be improved, more of what the student does well).

I have come to realize that, although there is some good to be found in the sandwich approach to providing feedback, this may contribute to the meat of the message being lost. When the student does not hear the true message, he or she cannot make the necessary adjustments for success. It is not caring to inhibit student progression toward goals. I now realize that sugarcoating the message is not equivalent to caring for my students. Rather, caring is demonstrated when a respectful tone within the context of trust is used to deliver a sometimes tough message.

Lesson 5: Preserve Student Dignity When Possible

Although I have seen several of my faculty colleagues adeptly use humor to address chatter in the room by drawing attention to it in front of the whole class, I have been dissatisfied with the results when I have attempted to target specific individuals publicly. They are often embarrassed and usually a vague uneasiness falls over the classroom. Some may argue that embarrassment is the price a student must pay for poor behavior. However, research suggests that students find public insults and humiliation to be unethical behavior on the part of faculty (Savage & Favret, 2006). Thus, I am not convinced the benefits outweigh the costs, especially when it can be avoided *and* results achieved.

I once had a challenging student who was frequently late turning in assignments and tardy for clinical experiences. During a conference with her to raise my concerns, I had already made one mistake by not addressing them earlier, she offered a multitude of excuses, and it was clear she would not be taking responsibility for her behavior any time soon. I made the decision to say something bold to coerce her into better behavior. "I am not here to be your babysitter," I remarked, hoping this comment would shame her into change. Unfortunately, her response was one of indignation, and she remained bitter and resentful the remainder of her time in our program. Although she presented ongoing challenges to our faculty, I regret that I used that approach. I actually apologized to her later, as it neither got the desired results nor buoyed my own self-perception.

In contrast, later in my career, I had a student who appeared to be involved in academic misconduct. After investigating, it appeared that this student had either knowingly or erroneously copied someone else's electronic files into her paper. During this incident, I remained objective, direct, and respectful in my interactions with her. Although the student received appropriate academic sanctions, she eventually went on to graduate and do well in her career. I continued to see this student as she completed our program and even now I occasionally see her in our community. There is no animosity that I can detect. I enjoy interacting with her, am proud of the contributions she makes to her workplace, and am glad to count her as a colleague.

Lesson 6: Help Them See How They May Be Affected

Giving constructive feedback is difficult at best. To get results, the student has to internalize the feedback. In the absence of internalization, it is tempting for the student to dismiss the feedback as arbitrary, suggesting that there is no valid reason to change behavior other than an instructor's whim. A key to ensuring that the feedback is internalized is to articulate how the behavior or performances affect the student. Perhaps more than any strategy I have employed when giving constructive feedback, this has been the most beneficial in achieving results. This can be attributed to two things. First, it demonstrates that you care about the student's well-being. Second, it takes the problem out of the instructor's lap and puts it in the lap of the student. Specifically, I use the following statements to help a student take ownership of a behavior and the ramifications of that behavior: "If you are okay with others potentially responding to you in this way (or drawing this conclusion about you), keep doing what you are doing, as it seems to be working. If, however, you are *not* okay with others potentially responding to you in this way (or drawing this conclusion about you), you may want to consider changing this particular behavior." Paramount to this lesson is the discernment between behaviors the student *must* change and behaviors the student should *consider* changing.

For example, once I had a student who chewed gum during her clinical experience with me on the floor. Additionally, she was vigorous in her mastication, so her chewing was visible and audible for some distance. Despite the fact that she was a fairly strong student, I found myself responding to her with consternation. I suspected that if I was responding to the gum chewing in a negative way, other professionals may as well. I had the option to tell her that our college rules prohibited her gum chewing, but this approach did not appeal to me because it did not require her to reflect critically on the impact of this seemingly benign behavior. Instead, I asked to speak to her privately about something I had noticed during her clinical rotation. I explained that, like it or not, people do form impressions of each other based on initial meetings. I shared with her that I was concerned that her gum chewing would potentially detract from all the good that she contributed to patient care because others might draw inaccurate conclusions about her professionalism. I also explained that since she was already appropriately proficient in her care delivery based on her level of learning, I was giving her feedback that would allow her to take her practice to an even higher level. I suggested that, if she wanted other health care workers to potentially draw the conclusion that she lacked professionalism, then she should keep on chewing gum in clinical. However, if she wanted to maximize her chances that others would view her as a professional, she might want to consider leaving her gum at home. In this case, I had to be prepared for the possibility that she would choose to continue her gum chewing.

This approach has been successful in dealing with student behavior related to sloppy dress, nonverbal communication, professional demeanor, and even performance on assignments. For example, when students turn in work that is not reflective of their true capability, I now take this approach. I tell students that I am left with two conclusions. Either in fact, they do not understand the material and are performing below par or they are someone who commits only partial effort to a task at hand. If indeed either of these conclusions is accurate and they are okay with me and others thinking that they lack understanding of the content or commit only half-heartedly to tasks at hand, by all means they should keep doing what they are doing because it is working. If, however, they want me and other people to conclude that they are committed individuals who apply themselves fully to the task at hand, they may want to consider changing their approach.

Lesson 7: Yes, Actually, We *Are* the Experts

Perhaps the single most emancipating lesson I have learned to date is this: I am an expert. In fact, it is my job to call on that expertise, and I am actually paid to do so. Ironically, this particular realization came by way of the especially unpleasant student mentioned in the introduction. I had been teaching about 3 years, still a novice in the higher education environment. After an exasperating semester of unpredictable clinical performance, inappropriate behavior, and second chances, it came time to deliver the news that she had not successfully met the course objectives, and thus had failed my class. In indignation, she responded, and I quote, "Who are you to decide this? You're not the expert you think you are!" At first speechless, I was tempted to consider this statement on its merit. Somewhere from the depth of my consciousness, however, an alternative explanation emerged. "Actually," I replied, "you are misinformed. I *am* an expert, and, in fact, it's my job to make judgments about your performance."

One of the most daunting aspects of the educator role is that of passing judgment on someone else's performance. The complexity associated with student evaluation is a common theme and the focal point of discussion innumerable times among my colleagues and faculty acquaintances. Unfortunately, it is virtually impossible to remove the subjective component from student evaluations, and it is that subjectivity that sometimes confounds our judgment. What if I have made a mistake? It is probably not a bad thing that those of us charged with passing judgment on others that may well affect the course of their lives should take pause.

However, assuming appropriate hiring practices, we are in educator roles because we have something to offer. We know nursing. We know what cognitive skills are required and what the appropriate behaviors are. More importantly, we know what nursing is not. Thus, when we have concerns about student behavior or student performance, our concerns most likely exist for a valid reason, even when we cannot articulate our concern. The challenge is to explore, identify, and ultimately articulate the underlying reason for the concerns.

Summary

The relationship between faculty and students is complex. Even those with formal training in education can be daunted by the task of shaping future nursing professionals. The reality is that many nursing faculty have little or no formal instruction in education. This situation can only exacerbate what is a common source of frustration for nurse educators: how to manage challenging student situations effectively. It is hoped that others may benefit from the mistakes made by this nurse educator and the subsequent lessons learned.

REFERENCES

American Nurses' Association. (2001). *Code of ethics for nurses with interpretive statements.* Washington, DC: American Nurses Publishing.

Lashley, F. R., & deMeneses, M. (2001). Student civility in nursing programs: A national survey. *Journal of Professional Nursing, 17*(2), 81–86.

Luparell, S. (2004). Faculty encounters with uncivil nursing students: An overview. *Journal of Professional Nursing, 20*(1), 59–67.

Luparell, S. (2005). Why and how we should address student incivility in nursing programs. In M. H. Oermann, & K. T. Heinrich, (Eds.), *Annual review of nursing education: Vol. 3. Strategies for teaching, assessment, and program planning* (pp. 23–36). New York: Springer Publishing.

National League for Nursing. (2002). Position statement on the preparation of nurse educators. *Nursing Education Perspectives, 23*(5), 267–269.

Savage, J. S., & Favret, J. O. (2006). Nursing students' perceptions of ethical behavior in undergraduate nursing faculty. *Nurse Education in Practice, 6,* 47–54.

Chapter 6

Investigating Women Nurse Academics' Experiences in Universities: The Importance of Hope, Optimism, and Career Resilience for Workplace Satisfaction

Nel Glass

A s nursing education becomes more diverse in approaches to learning, additional pressure and demands are exerted on academic faculty and clinicians to positively adopt and integrate new technological methods into their teaching portfolios. By way of example, information and communication technological enhanced learning, online course delivery, and wireless technology are now becoming expected rather than unique in university education (Billings, 2005). In general terms, it is imperative that faculty are preparing students to be exceedingly flexible, in both their approaches and expectations to education, to ensure learners take greater responsibility for their individual needs.

Although student-centered learning should be applauded, effective education undoubtedly does not occur in a vacuum and therein lays an educational impediment. Even though faculty acknowledge that diversity in teaching and learning, such as information and communication technology and online delivery, adds a richness to educational interactions (Morgan, Dunn, Parry, & O'Reilly, 2004), and student outcomes resulting in deep learning are desirable, achievements from such an

This chapter was accepted on December 18, 2005.

educational challenge require both flexibility and additional training. Furthermore, it is critical to acknowledge that, "teachers continue to struggle with how to best know and connect with students from a distance" (Diekelmann & Mendias, 2005, p. 344). Therefore faculty require both institutional support to adopt these educational developments and "on-the-ground" personnel and physical infrastructure support.

One could argue that faculty responding to this change in course delivery is an expected measure of career resilience and academic performance. Yet, when one delves into the reality of university workplace environments—specifically the current directions of universities—it is evident that faculty are constantly experiencing additional and competing demands on their time, and the aforementioned issue is just one example. Such a culture oftentimes results in faculty experiencing unrealistic pressure and stress; therefore, the introduction of further educational innovations is perceived negatively. Some faculty experience dialectical tension, wherein they are torn between their internal pressure to perform and external pressure to demonstrate competency among their peers and be positive to students.

Moreover, it is evident from the results of the study that follows that the management and organizational functioning of universities is fraught with difficulties. Faculty experience competing interpersonal and professional demands, and support for their own development remains at an all-time low. The issues at the forefront for faculty in schools of nursing are competitiveness, lack of support, bullying by faculty, and interpersonal violence. These issues directly affect academics' individual development and their ability to effectively take on new educational approaches such as those identified previously. A better understanding of university functioning and support of individual faculty is vital to the advancement and delivery of nursing education.

This chapter shares the experiences of women nurse academics who participated in a feminist, ethnographic study that involved four countries—(1) Australia, (2) New Zealand, (3) the United Kingdom, and (4) the United States—over an 8-year period (1997–2004). Highlighted are the competitive university cultures and the hope and optimism nurse academics desperately want to keep hold of. Their comments exposed a new emerging discourse of nurses in academia and revealed their interpersonal experiences of working in an academic setting. The major dominant features of these experiences are workplace violence and vulnerability.

The Challenge: Personal Motivation for the Study

I started my career in nursing education 30 years ago. Initially, I was employed as a nurse educator teaching in hospitals, and for the last 20 years I have been working as a nurse academic in universities. Although I have witnessed and experienced negativity and professional jealously in nursing education on several occasions, I have also held a strong belief that it was possible to do something positive about destructive behaviors in nursing. The literature for more than 2 decades has revealed "horizontal" violence (violence directed *at* colleagues working along side each other) in health care settings, which has not been evident in academic settings. Nurse academics have remained silent about their experiences of workplace violence. Therefore, I believed that more needed to be known of the experiences of women nurse academics nationally and internationally, and, to achieve this, nurses need to feel able to share their stories.

Background Literature

Current University Context

When considering large-scale organizations, it is evident that a culture of extensive budgetary restraint and institutional competitiveness, driven by financially motivated policy and decision-making, has become the new normal. Inherent within "work more for less" contexts where change is a constant, the escalating chronic pressures exerted on employees to excel at a fast pace and the inherent demands have resulted in decreased productivity, defensiveness, protracted stress, and burnout (Blonna, 2005; Gowing, Kraft, & Quick, 1998; Rose & Glass 2006; WFD Consulting, 2004).

In the main, public universities are in receipt of less governmental funding, and an increasing number of academics are expected to have strong outputs from income-generating activities. Moreover, greater rewards are assigned to those involved with scientific research pursuits. In contrast, lesser privileges are afforded to those academics employed in nonscientific disciplines (Department of Education, Science, and Training, 2004; Nelson, 2005; Roberts, 2003).

The dominant research discourses and agendas have resulted in environments filled with tension and ambivalence; those in professional and nonscientific disciplines, and in particular women, are experiencing limitations in their academic progression (Lee, 2004; Roberts & Turnbull, 2004). Decisions about how to "get on" and get ahead are directly linked to the political context of research activity such as the Research Assessment Exercise in the United Kingdom (UK), Performance-Based Research Fund in New Zealand (NZ), and Research Quality Frameworks being developed in Australia. The recognition that is afforded research active faculty, principally those with a strong research profile and outcomes of international significance, are now well entrenched into academics discourses internationally.

This notwithstanding, the dominance of research implies almost a nonevent with regard to other university responsibilities such as education. Teaching contracts, positions, and posts are not afforded the same significance as research, and as such are marginalized. Paradoxically, excellent teachers are just as necessary to the success and growth of universities, and attracting students is often directly linked to each university's reputation of excellence in teaching.

Yet, it is the fallout from these unrealistic pressures that are affecting women and nurses particularly. Decisions regarding whether to get on a tenure track, be research active, or be on a sole-teaching contract is significant to one's career. For women, the questions of career aspirations and political and social agendas that often include managing families are in direct opposition with university strategies and priorities (Lee, 2004). Nurses also have different research ideas and topics of interest from mainstream academia—most notably their professional stance and their evidenced-based practice research—and should be benchmarked accurately in terms of discipline specificity.

Both Usher (2004) and Nelson (2005) have argued for realistic discipline recognition. On behalf of the Australia and New Zealand Council of Deans of Nursing and Midwifery, Usher (2004) made a plausible case for a significant increase in the existing allocation of funds for qualitative nursing research, the method chosen by most nurses. The substance of Nelson's (2005) contention, in the response to the Australian government's Research Quality Framework issues paper, was for the discipline recognition based on the diversity of nurse academics activities. Nelson (2005) stated nurse academics needed to be recognized and measured alongside their peers by their engagement in journal publications, conference presentations and publication, and equally national and international peer esteem recognition, such as serving on editorial boards. Both Usher (2004) and Nelson (2005) have argued convincingly that it is not possible for nurses to be measured accurately by the major benchmarks of the scientific disciplines—those being large, competitive, national empirical grants achievements, bibliometrics, and citation indices in isolation.

Hence, nurse academics have argued for a level playing field across all academic disciplines and an explicit acknowledgment of the unique research that arises from those involved in practice-based disciplines (Australia & New Zealand Council of Deans of Nursing & Midwifery, 2005). Such a stance demonstrates evidence of political astuteness and emotional intelligence such that nurse academics are validating nursing as a discipline in the academy in its own right and as an equal university player.

Workplace Pressure and Health Issues

There is a plethora of literature that identifies stress and pressure as major health issues and argues for closely aligned personal and professional growth in efforts to reach workplace satisfaction (Caan, Morris, Santa Maria, & Brandon, 2000; Farrington, 1997; Giardano, Dusek, & Everly, 2005; Glass & Davis, 2004; Hall, 1997; Sherwood & Tager, 2002). Furthermore, we are warned about false splits between personal and career issues and the need to prioritize personal issues to ultimately improve career issues (Richardson, 1996). An integral theme is the emphasis on the relationship between achieving self-integration and personal well-being, and subsequent professional integration and satisfaction (Glass, 1997, 2003a; Hall, 1997; Lauver, 2000). The premise of this argument being, the more complete one is personally, the more complete one is professionally.

Personal and Professional Resilience

As a result of the increasing workplace organizational pressures, resilience and psychological well-being are now featured progressively more in the literature. For example, in response to the pace and ongoing change in the workplace, maintaining career resilience is determined more so by worker employability and associated flexibility than the out-dated notion of job security (Collard, Epperheimer, & Saign, 1996; Rick-wood, 2002). This has specific relevance for universities where, increasingly, appointments are contractual and not "continuing" nor tenured (Glass, 2003b, 2003c). In line with psychological growth, literature has defined career resilience as "the ability to adapt to changing circumstances, even when the circumstances are discouraging or disruptive" (Collard et al., 1996, p. 33). Career self-reliance is the degree to which one stays focused on one's own personal goals yet concurrently maintains an allegiance to workplace institutional goals. Furthermore, career resilience is integrally linked to career self-reliance where resilience is identified as the outcome of reliance (Collard et al., 1996).

Gillespie's (2005) recent study also informed this literature. Her research with Australian operating room nurses identified competence, knowledge, teamwork, social support, and situational control as critical aspects necessary to build resilience. What is critical is that employers and therefore institutional interpersonal relations have a role to play in employees developing resilience and subsequent intrapersonal work satisfaction.

Additionally, U.S. literature has directed greater attention to the need for resilience, particularly after the catastrophic events of 9/11. For example, in 2002, the American Psychological Association began to award organizations for specific policies, procedures and practices adopted to assist their employees build resilience (Business Wire, 2002). Although it is critical to acknowledge the aftermath of terrorist attacks and to ascertain the degree to which employees can work effectively under extremely difficult circumstances, supporting all employees in building resilience is a much broader issue. For instance, coping effectively at work among adversity is much more common; yet, there is a dearth of literature on the importance of resilience and workplace satisfaction in the absence of massive trauma. This does not deny that employers need to react to disaster by considering, maintaining, and sustaining resilience in the workplace. However, this begs the question: Why must employers wait for a disaster to consider the personal and professional growth and attributes of employees? Arguably a focus on resilience as a reaction to major events is socially and politically acceptable; yet, this is often in stark contrast to employers' attitudes to the "everydayness" of workplace demands.

Perhaps another way of perceiving resilience is that of "career responsiveness" suggested by Neault (2000). Neault (2000) claimed career responsiveness is a proactive stance and encompasses flexibility with environmental changes and being adaptable to internal needs. This has broader relevance for workplace institutions, irrespective of whether they are educational or health based, and as such plays a role in supporting the health of all workers.

Emotional Intelligence

Recent health-related literature refers to the notion of emotional intelligence (EI), a concept integrally linked to resilience (Edward & Warelow, 2005). Essentially, the literature reveals the need to focus on what nurses are doing in practice (Freshwater & Stickley, 2004), the role EI plays in forming successful human relationships, and for nursing leaders, the relationship to successful management (McQueen, 2004). Emotional intelligence is considered to be an asset in situations where it is important to understand other people, be an effective manager, and, in the main, consider the welfare of employees (Vitello-Cicciu, 2002). The EI challenge put forth is to look within oneself and "go to the heart of the art" (Freshwater & Stickley, 2004) and consider the concurrent impact of self-awareness and reflexive practice on the quality of staff and students' interactions.

What I Did: The Research Project

Research Aims

The aims of the research were to explore the following: participants' individual experiences and progression within their school of nursing and university; the specific sociopolitical contexts in which women nurse academics interact within both the school and university; the interpersonal relationships embedded within these cultures; to what extent participants were supported to progress and develop as scholars in their workplace; and what cultural and sociopolitical factors enhanced or inhibited their workplace achievements.

Research Design: Ethnography

The research was designed as a multisited "integrated feminist postmodern" study (Glass & Davis, 1998). Ethnography can be a method (Byrne, 2001), methodology (Manias & Street, 2001) or both, such that it can embody theoretical concepts and ideological practices (Berger, 1993; Walter, 2003). In terms of my selected theoretical constructs, feminist postmodern methodology was used to frame the ethnography and methods of data collection.

Contemporary ethnographers immersed in both the experiences and behaviors of those they are researching are significantly contrasted with the practices of traditional ethnographers who were expected to be distant observers (Richardson, 2000; Walter, 2003). Oftentimes, contemporary ethnographers are active, rather than passive, research participators, who simultaneously observe their culture under investigation. Therefore, as active researchers, they are extremely reliant on conversations that share and exchange lives, selves, and voices (Coffey, 1999). Ethnographers "draw close," and "this closeness to the practical ways people enact their lives" (Lather, 2001, p. 202) is critical to gain a comprehensive understanding of their participants. Yet, an equal challenge with undertaking a cross-cultural ethnography is the one posed by Crystal, a participant from NZ. She inquired: "How as an ethnographer do you choose the descriptors for people that fit within their own culture and how much of it is inevitably colored by your own?" Therefore, being open as a researcher and clarifying specific information to ensure it is accurately interpreted culturally is also a key aspect of this research.

Research Design: Feminist Postmodernism

Feminist framing acknowledges the epistemological belief that women are oppressed (Davis, 1998; Glass & Walter, 2000; Roberts, 2000) and offers emancipatory potential (Walter, Glass, & Davis, 2001). Postmodernism strengthens feminism in that it purports to acknowledge women's unique sociopolitical experiences within their particular context; validate difference and diversity of perceptions within that context; and recognize the impact of the "oppression narrative within each woman's 'everyday life' [by] creating opportunities to deconstruct their stories of experiences" (Glass, 2001a). Importantly, as Glass and Davis (1998) have argued, an integrated feminist postmodernism does not minimize the additional relevance of critical theory. Therefore, such theory acknowledges feelings of oppression that affect all women and equally takes into account the specific differences of life experiences for each individual woman.

The feminist construct of women finding voice and being heard (Heinrich, 2001; Walter et al., 2001) is a major factor in feminist ethnographies, and it is this particularly that creates and sustains the deeper interpersonal connection that can be achieved between the researcher and participants. Feminist postmodernism incorporates the desire to reclaim the totality of individual women's voices such that it valorizes the experiences of women (Glass, 1998; Ogle, 2004). Yet, one must heed the warning of Kane and Thomas (2000) that feminist postmodernism does not aim to locate one general voice, "the search for a coherent feminist nursing voice could lead us to silencing [all] voices" (p. 23).

Research Design: Methods

Three methods were used to triangulate the data, thereby affording greater strength to the study design (Denzin & Lincoln, 1998). The methods were participant observation, reflective journaling, and interviews.

Participant observation enabled a flexible level of involvement with each nurse educator. Therefore, as a researcher I could have a direct contribution in a role responsibility such as coteaching or conversely, a more passive involvement such as observation with concurrent reflection. Oftentimes, my involvement with each person was changeable, so that on one interaction, it may have been very active and the following one, much more silent and reflective.

Reflective journaling incorporating researcher intersubjectivity meant as a researcher I was deeply embedded in the research activities (Walter, Davis, & Glass, 1999). This method served two interwoven functions. It became a positive tool for my own therapeutic conversations (Glass, 2003b), and this was especially beneficial following observation of difficult workplace interactions. Equally, my journal was a field book in which I recorded specific observations and interpersonal interactions occurring at a specific time. Finally, the interviews were recorded over 1–2 hours toward the end of the time in each field. The first two methods served as triggers for the interviews and therefore enabled a further understanding of the conditions being studied (Downe, 1999).

Research Design: Ethics

Commenced in 1997 and completed in 2004, initial institutional ethical approval was gained for the research at the first institution. Over the course of the time of the ethnography, each university site made a further decision either to immediately approve the research or to forward the research proposal to their own university ethics committee. Following institutional ethics approval, participants were accessed initially via an introductory e-mail summarizing the project. The e-mail had two attachments: the information sheet and consent form. The e-mail was distributed to all school academics by my designated contact person in each country. Interested persons were then able to directly e-mail me, and I was then able to discuss the project most comprehensively and respond to any concerns about the nature and proposed progression of the project. Following signing of the consent forms, field data were collected.

What Did I Learn?

Biographical Data

Nine universities participated in the research across four countries: (1) Australia, (2) New Zealand, (3) the United Kingdom, and (4) the United States. Nearly half (47%) were from Australia (Figure 6.1). Of the 53 participants, 47% were lecturers, 17% were full professors, and 13% were associate professors; other ranks of participants are seen in Figure 6.2. Pseudonyms were assigned for each person; all identifying materials were altered to maintain anonymity, yet the substance of the disclosing information was retained. Moreover, in terms of participant confidentiality, at times, the country of the participant is identified; at other times, they are identified as either a Northern Hemisphere or Southern Hemisphere participant, or there is no reference to one's country or their workplace.

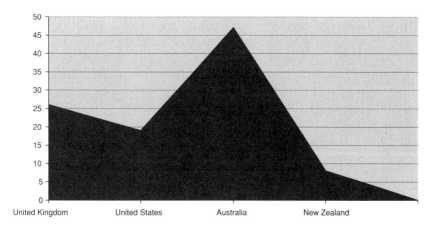

FIGURE 6.1   Participating countries and respective percentage of participants.

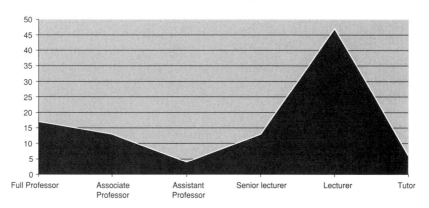

FIGURE 6.2   Academic rank of participants.

Work Context: Nurse Academics at Work

Results revealed participants were working for two entities: (1) their school of nursing and (2) the broader university. At times, the directions were in tandem; yet, oftentimes, they were at odds, resulting in the development of a counterculture. In most universities, nurses were treated as new and foreign in both their disciplinary approaches and research activities. Therefore, their plight was in stark contrast to university traditions, and this added to additional work pressures. Sorrell, a U.K. academic, confirmed these types of university observations and "top down" directions with this comment:

> Nursing is such a new discipline . . . each year that passes, there seems to be something new that's added to the things you have to put on your CV. . . . This particular institution is very [demanding] and that's not just in nursing, that's across the institution. The institution likes dictatorships.

Myfwany, an Australian academic, put it this way:

> [We] are learning on the hop and teaching it. I mean, I find that quite distressing because . . . you're not using peoples expertise and I guess, I think . . . it smacks of de-skilling and not valuing and it's all generating this sense of competitiveness all of which I find quite distasteful. An anathema really.

Although I would confirm that "academia remains a tough climate in which to work irrespective of discipline area" (Glass, 2003b, p. 180), the results indicated that nursing is seen as extraneous and problematic to many universities. The old adage of *publish or perish* in universities is not only upheld, but disadvantages nurses as they continue to be incorrectly benchmarked against the traditional scientists (Nelson, 2005). In conversation with Sorrell, she spoke of a university panel comprised of nursing and biological science academics that exemplified the disparate perceptions of nurse academics. She said nursing "wasn't considered up to the standard because it's just, the bio scientists are 'attracting.' They've just had huge investment, they are very strong . . . like the top . . . they are attracting real [dollars]."

In the schools of nursing, the culture was often very hostile and soul destroying. As Mikiala, an Australian academic, stated emphatically, "well it was like I was drowning." As her story unfolded, some of her professional challenges and successes, as well as her deep personal pain regarding the support of herself at the expense of other colleagues, became apparent. She related:

> Being in the [senior academic management] role gave me a different level of operation within the university. I went to different committees . . . there was a different, opportunity for me than existed when . . . I was Senior Lecturer. I got tenure really quickly. . . . I had a very more visible kind of a role.

She reflected on the treatment of her colleague who:

> was much more in the firing line [with] the university and [the Dean] than I ever was . . . . [She] just broke her heart over this place and still does. And she didn't get tenure for a long, long time and she didn't get tenure purely because of the Dean's vitriol you know! So for me to get tenure, everybody, including myself, was completely silent about it . . . . We all felt devastated about all of that and powerless because we knew that the enemy was not the university, the enemy was [the Dean] . . . . He blocked her because she, she had this 'voice' . . . when you know that what you're doing is going to rebound on you . . . but you have to do it anyway because it comes from your soul . . . it's like [the Dean] sets someone up to do everything, sets this absolutely impossible task and then when you can't do it because it was always impossible, it's to do with your personal lack of ability.

Yet for some participants their school culture had improved, yet as Crystal said, it was still necessary to be sure how and in what ways to interact with colleagues. She put it this way:

> I still feel I can say what I want to say. It's just finding the space to step into. Yeah! I wonder if it's . . . an echo of what it was like when I first came [to the school] . . . and it felt to me at the time like I was encountering a siege mentality . . . at the time it felt like you were absolutely the new person and you don't understand how things are and even if you learned about it, you'd still get it wrong, and very much unable to offer anything.

Furthermore, as many nurse academics in the UK, Australia, and NZ were also gaining their own research qualifications while being concurrently involved in additional research projects and carrying a substantial teaching load, the academic pressure was very strong (Glass, 2001a, 2001b; Worrall-Carter & Snell, 2003). Moreover, disciplines with high concentrations of women are affected extensively. For instance, in Australia, women remain concentrated at the bottom of the academic hierarchy with only 20% of associate professors and full professors being women (Carrington & Pratt, 2003).

Consequently, women nurse academics have difficulty feeling hopeful about their university career and for some they cannot perceive it is possible to be optimistic about their future. In Sunny's words: "There is still a period of feeling very down about 'tomorrow'." In terms of hope, she questioned: "It's galvanizing that energy really, isn't it?"

As Tess, a Southern Hemisphere academic, said of the head of her school:

> I have a fundamental distrust.... I am finding it extremely difficult and it has had an impact right through the whole school.... I see a pattern with [her]... it is a highly developed pattern of manipulation where she will talk about other [faculty]... she does not lead, it's just control.

Moreover, as Pearl put it, being a senior woman academic in a male-dominated university positions one to be perceived as token. She explained: "the downside... there's also the danger of being promoted onto committees and those sorts of things and I'm sometimes asked am I here because I'm the token female or am I here because of what I can contribute."

Additionally, like Siler and Kleiner (2001), I found that support within schools was not necessarily forthcoming for individual nurses, and novice faculty were the main sufferers. As has been written earlier, some interactions among nurses were hostile, volatile, and violent. Disturbingly, support, recognition, and validation were minimal, and it was clear that their quest to get on in the university culture was often directly hampered by their own faculty, as well as by the broader university (Glass, 2003b, 2003c; Glass & Davis, 2004; Roberts, 1997; Roberts & Turnbull, 2004).

Some participants attributed these destructive behaviors to a relocation of the hospital culture of nursing. Isis spoke of horizontal violence and bullying and confirmed its occurrence. She stated emphatically:

> Definitely! And the problem with that is,... we've all come through the NHS [National Health Service] which was run like the army when I trained.... And you were trained not to challenge, not to ask questions, to accept. And so that kind of pervasive way of thinking doesn't just stop. Unfortunately it's still, still alive.

Sarah reasoned: "I think it is a symptom of nursing... the stuff we 'get' at the university is all like extensions of what really goes on in nursing." Yet, for a few, there was support in specific areas of their school of nursing but not others.

Leigh revealed her contrasting positive and negative experiences:

> If I put an idea out on the table or any body else did... you wouldn't pounce on it, you would look at it and say you know, well I can take this, and see it through... it was all about... nurturing and supporting/helping to grow. [Whereas] the opposite you'd put an idea on the table and you'd get a 1000

reasons why it wouldn't work or what was wrong with it, what was stupid about it, such that I would never talk about what I tried in the classroom, what I was thinking about something, you know, because it was not a place to be comfortable . . . on any dimension. It was not fair play, you always got pounced.

Another way of illustrating this volatility was expressed by Lauren, a senior NH nurse academic. She spoke of her intolerance for novice academics becoming acculturated:

I have little patience to shut up in meetings where people are talking about 'well, I'm very new at this and we have to look at our profile'. . . [this] lets learn how to do academia business you know. I think well, you're here so you should do it, you know like everybody else.

Competitiveness within schools was also manifested by lack of support for professional development, and as a consequence a growing isolation was experienced. For instance, it was repeatedly confirmed there is limited or no professional drive, nor support from other nurse academics, and the academic herself or himself has to be the "driver." For instance, Sarah, who made a decision to leave academia, believed if she expected support from others: "I'd still be a staff nurse . . . maybe I've never really had support. I don't think people really know where I'm coming from . . . . I occasionally have a bit of encouragement and I've occasionally been given a bit of insight [from a non nurse]."

Similar experiences were voiced by Bloddwyn, a U.K. academic: "It's the professional thing that is the problem . . . because [the school of nursing] doesn't have any. The one thing that I find the most difficult is the waste of individual talent. . . . I don't really have any kind of professional [fulfillment]."

University restructures and subsequent school changes were also identified as causes of personal and professional isolation. Sunny reflected on losing teaching teams and any sense that nursing education has a bearing in her university. She said:

The management has changed and that has taken away the team completely, it doesn't exist anymore . . . now we're just on our own. . . . I've been thinking . . . in the four or five years that we've been in the university, how badly behaved many of the managers are. They do a knee-jerk reaction and don't actually justify many of the decisions. . . . There is a lack of value in education. There is a lack of appreciation and value of the skill.

Sunny also spoke of isolation in the context of professional performance review:

> [My manager] was looking at my last performance review. . . . There is no
> feedback from the university. It's all about "what did I think?" . . . there's no
> comment from your . . . manager as to how you're doing. It is one way. . . .
> I'm not saying that I should be nursed and carried or people should do it
> all for me, but it doesn't appear to be anything being offered from the other
> way. . . . I don't feel it's supported. . . . I feel it's very much, go out and fight
> for what you can get.

Resilience and Importance of the "Person"

It was indisputable that adaptation to the constancy of changes within both the university in totality and the schools placed undue pressure on many participants. Above all, the stress participants felt tested them as people, and explicitly, the ways in which they reacted to work priorities. This was most obvious as participants attempted to progress their careers. Their efforts resulted in vulnerability, stress, and burnout, necessitating active healing interventions and strategies (Glass, 1997, 2003a).

Robyn, a U.K. academic, believed that those managing nursing and the university have little time for the humanness of their faculty. She reflected:

> . . . they feel uncertain about passionate people. . . . We've gone through sev-
> eral amalgamations, different schools, different cultures as well, and I think
> that we've grown to [3 times larger] and I think that it's a big sense of loss its
> alien to what I believe—I believe that I'm a people person. And [now] people
> don't take time I don't think to get to know people at all. That isn't there,
> there isn't a means or framework, in the school, to bring people together,
> so whereas . . . we [used to] debate until our hearts content and we would
> laugh and all those wonderful human activities, and now it's like we're little
> rats, behind the door, and nobody knows you're there.

Participants spoke of the importance of their resilience, autonomy, self-reliance and confidence to interface their workplace. They were aware that career resilience, essential to cope effectively with adversity, was an important component of their university survival (Dyer & McGuinness, 1996). As Ronel said: "It depends on the person. To survive . . . I think you have to be quite strong in yourself and determine where you are going. . . . You have to learn to set your boundaries."

It was evident that positive constructs—such as hope, optimism, and resilience—were critical to the participants' professional satisfaction, emotional well-being, and professional outcomes (Glass, 2001b; Glass & Davis, 2004) as was a conscious revisioning of their world views (Glass, 2003a). There were integral links between recognizing and attempting to let go of vulnerability by acknowledging hope and resilience within self. Having and/or regaining a belief in themselves and if possible, their colleagues contributed significantly to a greater perception of their workplace (Glass, 2003a). As Wyn, a U.S. academic said: "I believe that everybody has their story and has something to offer. . . . I think that people have pretty legitimate ideas . . . and have something to offer and are well intentioned."

The participants consciously chose to invert the negatively constructed vulnerability as weakness, by moving through vulnerability to an empowered positive position that enhanced personal and professional outcomes (Glass & Davis, 2004). Such recognition decreased stress and created a therapeutic freeing (Glass & Davis, 2004; Hem & Heggen, 2003).

Therapeutic freeing in this context implies participants were able to reach out to colleagues who were supportive of their situation and verbalize positive ways of reframing their workplace. Therefore, they were psychologically mobilizing and releasing their negative emotions and perceptions, as well as developing emotional intelligence—both notions considered essential to their survival in a nursing faculty. Moreover, if their vulnerability was cognitively reframed as a positive concept (Glass & Davis, 2004), it was possible for participants to become hopeful about their workplace. Lin, a Northern Hemisphere academic, put it like this: "I try to be mindful of my relationships with others and hopefully there is a feeling of mutual respect. . . . I work on the inner calm."

By actions such as these, participants experienced initially a sense of relief that they have finally spoken about destructive workplace practices without judgment, and in the longer term, they gained a belief and inner strength to continue to disclose and enhance their sense of self. Ultimately, this led to a greater sense of knowing self and hence personal and professional integration. On the contrary, if these values were not supported, satisfaction in employment and productivity were hindered.

Isis reflected on her revisioning and hope in her actions at the university:

> I tend to gravitate toward those people who are women sensitive in their approach to care, but really give a damn about . . . what we should be

doing and what we're not doing. . . . [After] I hit the water . . . I didn't give a damn anymore about the things that I used to feel were really important like relying on other people for your success or . . . happiness . . . you are responsible for yourself . . . you've got to do it yourself, so in that you've then got to take responsibility. . . . I actively seek out positive people and I actively avoid negative people. . . . I feel that I am very intuitive in the sense that it's something that developed over the years of being a nurse and midwife . . . so if I do have to deal with negative people, [I do not] actually get down.

Sarah actively incorporated an optimistic approach to work by cognitively revisioning her thoughts. She shared:

The way I say it is: what will make me feel better? What can I get out of this? How can I stop feeling like this? And what is it I can do now to make me feel better? What will help me to get on? And how can I feel happier about this situation? You know, there is no good being a victim to it, what can you do to make it better? You've got loads of things you can do, so go and do something.

Cerridwen, a Northern Hemisphere academic, revisioned her workplace to be perceived optimistically by generosity. She reflected on an interaction at work:

I was determined to make it work, from my perspective of course because I wanted it to, . . . and I felt I was quite generous in meeting the requirements of the job, in fact I was beyond that really, which is part of the generosity I suppose . . . but it's not always the way other people are back too, and I'm not doing it so people will reciprocate. I guess because I always look at the collective and think that if we all kind of work together and accommodate each other and do this and that will make for a better environment.

For Bloddwyn, her colleagues' respect and acknowledgement contributed to her career resilience.

Yet all I want is somebody actually utilizing my strengths and saying thanks. . . . That's all I want, I don't want anything else. Like the Dean saying to me 'like I love the way you deal with students. . . . I couldn't have done it without you, I want you to do it again.' That's it, that's all I need. . . . And that's utilizing my professional talents. . . . It means utilizing me in a way that's good for them and good for me and valuing that and not diminishing what's there. It doesn't necessarily mean getting my own way all the time, or me having total freedom.

What Does This Mean? Implications for Nurse Educators

Challenge of Instilling Hope for Academics and Their Workplace

Although participants spoke of hope, it was evident that there were inherent challenges in being able to instill and sustain it. Yet, this was deemed necessary to become professionally satisfied as individual academics and regain workplace satisfaction. Seemingly, hope was perceived as an essential component of resilience, and personal and career resilience were integral to well-being. Moreover, in a cyclical manner, personal and professional well-being had resulted in feelings of empowerment/empowered states, professional satisfaction, and integration; in turn, optimism was able to be manifested if participants were hopeful and resilient (Glass, 1998; Glass & Davis, 2004; Hochswender, Martin, & Morino, 2001; Russinova, 1999).

Therefore, this implies that whereas resilience requires an ability to be future orientated, hope and optimism cannot occur for nurse educators without a cognitive reframing and revisioning concerning the possibility that one can have an optimistic future at work. As this research has shown—if nurse educators had hopeful and optimistic thoughts, feelings, and actions—their levels of resilience would increase and, most importantly, if utilized, professional satisfaction could result.

One of the challenges in education concerns the need to manage stress and improve well-being at work. Undoubtedly, nurse academics who speak of hope and resilience need to be heard and supported consistently by their educational colleagues and managers. All participants had strong ideas about how, and in what ways, their school of nursing could become a more positive place to work. Yet, participants ideas were in fact not heard and their beliefs about hope and optimism in the workplace were actually minimized.

Therefore, although it is critical to be hopeful and optimistic, if their thoughts and actions are curtailed, nurses lose their hope and passion for nursing education. For instance, this challenge was obvious in Leigh's story, a U.S. academic, when she spoke of her attempts to perceive her colleagues more positively in the face of destructive behaviours. Leigh related an experience at a faculty retreat where she attempted to cognitively reframe her view of some of her faculty. In particular, she questioned was there any possibility of collegial reconciliation. Leigh said:

.... we spent many, many days in retreats... [and] for the first time a few people around the table really kind of dropped down their shield at bit and we started to be known as people.... I can remember sitting there talking myself into saying, I can care about these people. I can see them now as people, maybe there is a way we can get past it... because I now know more about them as people. But, that didn't last very long. You know I was really kind of persuading myself, that because I had seen a glimpse of them at a personal level that I could sort of let a lot of the other stuff go that somehow it made it forgivable—the violence stuff [but] what they were doing in front of me, but it really wasn't forgivable stuff.

Disturbingly Leigh's experience was representative of most of the participants. The need for positive practices and ways of thinking to be utilized in academic practices was forefront in the minds of participants, yet such ideas were more like dreams than their reality. Therefore, hope, resilience, and optimism were marginalized and, as such, were subjugated discourses in their academic life (Glass & Davis, 2004). Nonetheless, "whilst emotional resilience was achieved by some participants this occurred over an extensive period of time and only came about if there was cultural change or emotional safety to speak out" (Glass & Davis, 2004, p. 89). Emotional safety was not a common event. Those who attempted to revise and incorporate positive cultural change were relegated to an "other" status and their workplaces remained unchanged.

Essentials for Improving Workplaces

I would strongly argue it is critical for nurse educators to continually reflect on their personal and career resilience and the degree to which self-reliance plays a role in their professional satisfaction. This is imperative because the impersonal relations in higher education constantly challenge and test individual faculty to react to decisions that seem to be heartless. It does require a very strong internal drive. As Crystal confirmed:

Well, if I put my mind to doing something, I do it. I do achieve. [Although] It's been hard being in any place where I've worked. It's just how I am.... I've had tremendous support from people outside of the discipline, outside of nursing... and that is hugely validating for me; that is like being accepted by my peers in another discipline and its just tremendous!

Moreover, academics need intrapersonal strength and professional resilience to reach and maintain workplace fulfillment, particularly because disclosing their lived passionate academic experiences is risky (Heinrich, 2001). Institutional oppression and competing university directions remain very powerful opposing forces. Such force is imposing and threatening and is consistently evidenced in workplaces. Academics have been shocked, angered, and disillusioned by their experiences of being unheard and unsaid (Glass, 2003c), and this is especially so when they have spoken out about creative workplace change. Unsurprisingly, teachers of nursing are at risk of upending their love and passion of education and research and leaving their chosen career. Notwithstanding this, nurses' voices can be strong and threatening such that, it is imperative that nurses are able to verbalize their stories to turn oppressive workplaces around.

Previous research has shown that nurses can be passionate about their career and become heroic in their educational approaches (Heinrich, 1997). Nurses need to weigh up the risks associated with keeping the status quo or voicing their stories (Heinrich, 2001). I would propose these strategies are deliberate, constructive, achievable ways to challenge the minimization of nurses' hopes for career improvement.

Above all, nurses need to reflect on and recognize their own personal strength and endurance in their workplace. It is important that nurses use strategies such as their own emotional intelligence and seek support from colleagues who are "there" for each other. This further builds personal resilience and in turn assists in additional strengthening of one's career resilience. Moreover, it is important to be aware that, while resilience requires the ability to bounce back from disturbing experiences, maintenance of strong professional boundaries regarding what faculty will take on in their workplace, along with EI, improves resilience.

Furthermore, it is imperative to reject the notion that workplaces as positive places to be are just rhetoric or impossible dreams. Nurses need a strong, collective commitment to reinvent their workplaces as positive, and this involves a philosophical shift so that this may result (Glass, 2003a; Glass & Davis, 2004; Heinrich, 2001). Valuing the inherent healer and intuitive ability within all nurses and midwives (Hemsley, Glass, & Watson, 2006; Hemsley & Glass, 2006) is critical to the adoption of a healing philosophy, and essential to managing destructive workplaces such as universities. Therefore, focusing on healing oneself and maintaining an inner calm should be upheld as critical strategically (Glass, 2003a). In terms of collegial interpersonal relations, being able to think in diverse and different ways to manage a new or old nursing problem requires valuing others' creativity in thinking, expression, storying, and academic ability to turn in and positively remake and reframe our working lives (Frank, 2003).

Conclusion

In summary, nurse educators need a positive professional perspective. It is not possible to work well and maintain our health without such a perspective. Work, although not everything in one's life, takes up a significant amount of time. Therefore, nurse educators are worthy and deserving of quality workplace interactions. Furthermore, it is critical that nurses acknowledge and celebrate the depth of their own intrapersonal strength because this is a significant indicator of personal and professional abilities. Moreover, nurses' resilience has enabled them to reach where they are now. *Yet, isn't that we want to nurture, protect, and value—such a precious ability to strengthen nurses and the profession now and beyond?* If this is so, it is overdue to seriously presence ourselves and really listen to ourselves and each other. It is this that brings further hope to nursing education.

Acknowledgements

The author acknowledges the participants who willingly gave of their time and shared, at times, very difficult experiences in support of nursing research. The author also acknowledges Southern Cross University, Australia, for funding this project.

REFERENCES

Australia and New Zealand Council of Deans of Nursing and Midwifery. (2005). *Research quality framework: Response to the issues paper*, Australian Government, Department of Education, Science and Training, March (Unpublished paper).

Berger, R. A. (1993). From text to (field) work and back again: Theorizing a post (modern)-Ethnography. *Anthropological Quarterly*, *66*, 174–186.

Billings, D. (2005). From teaching to learning in a mobile, wireless world. *Journal of Nursing Education*, *44*, 343.

Blonna, R. (2005). *Coping with stress in a changing world* (3rd ed.). New York: McGraw Hill.

Business Wire. (2002). *Companies honored for psychologically healthy workplace practices: American Psychological Association recognizes resilient workplaces*. September 26, 2002. Retrieved July 15, 2005, from http://www.businesswire.com

Byrne, M. (2001). Ethnography as a qualitative research method. *AORN Online*, *74*(1), 82–84.

Caan, W., Morris, L., Santa Maria, C., & Brandon, D. (2000). Wounded healers. *Nursing Standard, 15*(2), 22–23.

Carrington, K., & Pratt, A. (2002–2003). How far have we come? Gender disparities in the Australian higher education system. *Current Issues Brief, 31*. Retrieved July 5, 2005, from www.une.edu.au/arts/Sociolog/STAFF/kcarrington.html

Coffey, A. (1999). *The ethnographic self: Fieldwork and the representation of identity*. London: Sage Publications, Inc.

Collard, B., Epperheimer, J. W., & Saign, D. (1996). *Career resilience in a changing workplace*. Columbus, OH: ERIC Clearinghouse on Adult, Career, and Vocational Education. (ED 396 191).

Davis, K. (1998). *Cartographies of rural community nursing and primary health care: Mapping the in-between spaces,* PhD Thesis. Hawkesbury, Australia: UWS-H.

Department of Education, Science, and Training (DEST). (2004). *Research quality framework: Consultation discussion starter*. Retrieved May 16, 2005, from Australian Government Web site http://www.dest.gov.au/resqual/#1

Denzin, N., & Lincoln, Y. (1998). *Strategies in qualitative inquiry*. Thousand Oaks CA: Sage Publications, Inc.

Diekelmann, N., & Mendias, E. (2005). Being a supportive presence in online courses: Knowing and connecting with students through writing. *Journal of Nursing Education*, *44*, 344–346.

Downe, P. (1999). Laughing when it hurts: Humour and violence in the lives of Costa Rican prostitutes. *Women's Studies International Forum, 22*(1), 63–78.

Dyer, J. G., & McGuinness, T. M. (1996). Resilience: Analysis of the concept. *Archives of Psychiatric Nursing*, *10*(5), 276–282.

Edward, K., & Warelow, P. (2005). Resilience: When coping is emotionally intelligent. *Journal of American Psychiatric Nurses Association*, *11*(2), 101–102.

Farrington, A. (1997). Strategies for reducing stress and burnout in nursing. *British Journal of Nursing, 6*(1), 44–50.

Frank, A. (2003). How stories remake what pain unmakes. In J. Dostrovsky, D. Carr, & M. Koltzenburg (Eds.), *Proceedings of the 10th World Congress on Pain, Progress in Pain Research and Management* (Vol. 24, pp. 619–630). Seattle: IASP Press.

Freshwater, D., & Stickley, T. (2004). The heart of the art: Emotional intelligence in nurse education. *Nursing Inquiry*, *11*(2), 91–98.

Gillespie, B. (2005). Predictors of resilience among operating room nurses. *Connections*, *8*(2), 30.

Giardano, D., Duskek, D., & Everly, G. S. Jr. (2005). *Controlling stress and tension* (7th ed.). San Francisco: Pearson.

Glass, N. (1997). Horizontal violence in nursing: Celebrating conscious healing strategies. *Australian Journal of Holistic Nursing, 4*(2), 15–23.

Glass, N. (1998). Becoming de-silenced and reclaiming voice: Women nurses speak out. In H. Keleher & F. McInerney (Eds.), *Nursing matters* (pp. 121–138). Melbourne: Churchill Livingstone.

Glass, N. (2001a). The dis-ease of nursing academia: Putting the vulnerability 'out there.' Part one. *Contemporary Nurse, 10*(3–4), 172–177.

Glass, N. (2001b). The dis-ease of nursing academia: Putting the vulnerability 'out there.' Part two. *Contemporary Nurse, 10*(3–4), 178–186.

Glass, N. (2003a). Validating moving on: Reflections of women nurse academics experiences with violence and subsequent healing. *Women Against Violence, 13,* 49–58.

Glass, N. (2003b). Studying women nurse academics: Exposing workplace violence. Part one. *Contemporary Nurse, 14*(2), 180–186.

Glass, N. (2003c). Studying women nurse academics: Exposing workplace violence. Part two. *Contemporary Nurse, 14*(2), 187–195.

Glass, N., & Davis, K. (1998). An emancipatory impulse: A feminist postmodern integrated turning point in nursing research. *Advances in Nursing Science, 21*(1), 43–52.

Glass, N., & Davis, K. (2004). Reconceptualizing vulnerability: Deconstruction and reconstruction as a postmodern feminist analytical research method. *Advances in Nursing Science, 27*(2), 82–92.

Glass, N., & Walter, R. (2000). An experience of peer mentoring with student nurses: Enhancement of personal and professional growth. *Journal of Nursing Education, 39*(4), 1–6.

Gowing, M. K., Kraft, J. D., & Quick, J. C. (1998). *The new organizational reality: Downsizing, restructuring, revitalization.* Washington, DC: American Psychological Association.

Hall, J. (1997). Nurses as wounded healers. The journey to healing the person and the profession. *Australian Journal of Holistic Nursing, 4*(1), 11–16.

Heinrich, K. (1997). Transforming imposters into heroes. *Nurse Educator, 22*(3), 45–50.

Heinrich, K. (2001). Doctoral women as passionate scholars: An exploratory inquiry of passionate dissertation scholarship. *Advances in Nursing Science, 23*(3), 88–103.

Hem, M., & Heggen, K. (2003). Being professional and being human: One nurse's relationship with a psychiatric patient. *Journal of Advanced Nursing, 43*(1), 101–108.

Hemsley, M.(S.), & Glass, N. (2006). Sacred journeys of nurse healers. *Journal of Holistic Nursing.* In press.

Hemsley, M., Glass, N., & Watson, J. (2006). Taking the eagle's view: Using Watson's conceptual model to investigate the extraordinary and transformative experiences of nurse healers. *Holistic Nursing Practice, 20*(2), 85–94.

Hochswender, W., Martin, G., & Morino, T. (2001). *The buddha in your mirror: Buddhism the search for self.* Santa Monica CA: Middleway Press.

Kane, D., & Thomas, B. (2000). Nursing and the "F" word. *Nursing Forum, 35*(2), 17–24.

Lather, P. (2001). Postbook: Working the ruins of feminist ethnography. *Signs, 27*(1), 199–230.

Lauver, D. R. (2000). Commonalities in women's spirituality and women's health. *Advances in Nursing Science, 22*(3), 76–88.

Lee, A. (2004). Research dilemmas for women in universities: Issues of strategy and *'worthwhileness.'* Perth, Western Australia: Curtin University of Technology.

Manias, E., & Street, A. (2001). Rethinking ethnography: Reconstructing nursing relationships. *Journal of Advanced Nursing, 33*(2), 234–242.

McQueen, A. (2004). Emotional intelligence in nursing work. *Journal of Advanced Nursing, 47*(1), 101–108.

Morgan, C., Dunn, L., Parry, S., & O'Reilly, M. (2004). *The student assessment handbook: New directions in traditional and online assessment.* London: Routledge Falmer.

Neault, R. (2000). Planning for serendipity? *Career management for changing times.* NATCON papers. Canada: Simon Fraser University. Retrieved October 14, 2005, from http://www.onestep.on.ca/resource/files2/Career%20Management%20for%20Changing%20Times.pdf

Nelson, S. (2005, February). *Research quality framework for Australian universities briefing paper: Background and implications* (2nd ed.). Melbourne: Council of Australian and New Zealand Deans of Nursing and Midwifery.

Ogle, K. R. (2004). *Shifting (com)positions on the subject of management: A critical feminist and postmodern ethnography of critical care nursing.* PhD Thesis, Lismore, Australia: Southern Cross University.

Richardson, M. (1996). From career counselling to counselling/psychotherapy and work, jobs, and career. In M. L. Savickas & W. B. Walsh (Eds.), *Handbook of career counselling theory and practices* (pp. 347–360). Palo Alto, CA: Davies-Black.

Richardson, L. (2000). Evaluating ethnography. *Qualitative Inquiry, 6*(2), 253–255.

Rickwood, R. (2002). *Enabling high-risk clients: Exploring a career resiliency model.* British Columbia, Canada: Nuu-Chah-nulth Tribal Council. Retrieved October 14, 2005, from http://www.contactpoint.ca/natcon-conat/2002/pdf/pdf-02-10.pdf

Roberts, G. (2003). *Review of research assessment for RA review—Joint funding bodies.* Retrieved May 16, 2005, from http://www.ra-review.ac.uk/reports/roberts.aspir

Roberts, K. (1997). Nurse academics' scholarly productivity: Framed by the system, facilitated by mentoring. *Australian Journal of Advanced Nursing, 14*(3), 5–14.

Roberts, K., & Turnbull, B. (2004). Nurse academics' scholarly productivity: Perceived frames and facilitators. *Contemporary Nurse 17* (3), 282–292.

Roberts, S. J. (2000). Development of a positive professional identity: Liberating oneself from the oppressor within. *Advances in Nursing Science, 22*(4), 71–82.

Rose, J., & Glass, N. (2006). Women community mental health nurses speak out: The critical relationship between emotional wellbeing and professional practice. *Collegian, 13*(4), 27–32.

Russinova, Z. (1999). Providers' hope-inspiring competence as a factor optimizing psychiatric rehabilitation outcomes. *Journal of Rehabilitation, 65*(4), 50–57.

Sherwood, P., & Tagar, Y. (2002). Philophonetics counselling for prevention of burnout in nurses. *Australian Journal of Holistic Nursing, 9*(2), 32–40.

Siler, B., & Kleiner, C. (2001). Novice faculty: Encountering expectations in academia. *Journal of Nursing Education, 40*, 397–403.

Usher, K. (2004). *Post election briefing paper.* Melbourne: Council of Deans of Nursing and Midwifery (Australia and New Zealand).

Vitello-Cicciu, J. M. (2002). Exploring emotional intelligence: Implications nursing leaders. *Journal of Nursing Administration, 32*(4), 203–210.

Walter, R. (2003). *Having the light attitude: An integrated postmodern feminist investigation of women graduate registered nurses and playfulness.* PhD thesis. Lismore, Australia: Southern Cross University.

Walter R., Davis, K., & Glass, N. (1999). Discovery of self: Exploring, interconnecting and integrating self (concept) and nursing. *Collegian, 6*(2), 12–16.

Walter, R., Glass, N., & Davis, K. (2001). Epistemology at work: The ontological relationship between feminist methods, intersubjectivity and nursing research—A research exemplar. *Contemporary Nurse, 10*(3–4), 265–272.

WFD Consulting. (2004). *When the going gets tough: Does your workforce have the resilience to keep going? It's about time.* Retrieved May 15, 2005, from http://www.wfd.com/news/past_news.html

Worrall-Carter, L., & Snell, R. (2003). Nurse academics meeting the challenges of scholarship and research. *Contemporary Nurse, 16*(1–2), 40–50.

Chapter 7

From Dancing With Hurricanes to Regaining Our Balance: A New Normal

Gwen Leigh, Jill Laroussini, Sudha C. Patel, and Ardith L. Sudduth

D ifficult and stressful do not even begin to describe what we— faculty and students at the University of Louisiana at Lafayette— endured during the fall semester of 2005. Hurricane Katrina hit the Gulf Coast of Louisiana, Mississippi, and Alabama on August 29, 2005. In preparation for the incoming hurricane, our university closed for 3 days. Hurricane Katrina was one of the most destructive storms to ever hit the United States, causing extensive damage. Levees protecting the city of New Orleans were breached, and 80% of this major city flooded. As a result of the storm, more than 1.5 million people were displaced, many to Lafayette. The area of destruction covered 90,000 square miles along the Gulf Coast, an area almost the size of the United Kingdom (Department of Homeland Security, 2005). Four weeks later, Hurricane Rita hit the Louisiana Gulf Coast, west of Lafayette, Louisiana. Again, our University closed down. Geographically sandwiched between two major hurricanes in 1 month, we all have many stories to tell about how we danced with these hurricanes and regained our balance in a new normal—not once but twice.

This chapter describes how the authors, four committed nurse ed-ucators on the University of Louisiana at Lafayette faculty, responded to a state of crisis while maintaining academic commitments, helping students to cope, and managing their own personal challenges created

This chapter was accepted on April 5, 2006.

137

by these storms. Jill Laroussini's section tells the story of how she balanced resourcefulness and flexibility while maintaining academic commitments. Sudha Patel and Ardith Sudduth's section shows how they helped students to cope. Gwen Leigh's section reviews how faculty managed their own personal challenges. Tips for nurse educators facing crises are taken from the lessons learned from Hurricanes Katrina and Rita.

A Classroom Story: Finding the New Normal

In this section, Jill Laroussini speaks to the challenge of maintaining academic integrity in the aftermath of the hurricanes. Our governor had declared a state of emergency following the largest natural disaster to hit our nation. Entering the classroom 3 days after Hurricane Katrina hit the Gulf Coast was not "business as usual." The signs of suffering were everywhere: in the eyes of the students, in the voices heard in the hallways, and in my heart and soul. While sitting in the safety of my living room, I had watched the growing red vortex called Katrina on the television screen as the huge storm moved inland. Sitting alongside me was my sister and her family who had evacuated New Orleans 2 days prior to the storm's landfall. We both knew at 10 a.m., without having to use any words, that our family home on the Mississippi Gulf Coast was nothing more than a concrete slab, just as it was when my parents built on it after Hurricane Camille. A youngster in the aftermath of Hurricane Camille, I witnessed the resourcefulness of my mother and two older brothers who delivered food and supplies to my relatives on the Mississippi Gulf Coast following the chaos and carnage left behind by that storm.

Now, 37 years later, it was my turn to contribute as a resourceful adult to the relief efforts. I believe that my past experiences prepared me for this moment and for the challenges to come. It was no coincidence that I had been learning about the new brain research on trauma, posttraumatic stress disorder (PTSD), and mind-body approaches to healing trauma (Naparstek, 2004) in preparation for the homecoming of our soldiers from Iraq. As a community nurse and chapter leader of a nonprofit organization that exists to help bridge the allopathic and complementary approaches to health and wellness, I had cocreated "Ready 4 the Return." Intended to empower families of soldiers with information about PTSD and the complementary path to recovery outside of traditional psychotherapy, "Ready 4 the Return" is a national community initiative of the Wholistic Wellness Network, Inc., that offers information about mind-body skill sets effective in healing trauma. Seeing the signs of trauma among us, I could see how these new skills might contribute to our healing.

My clinical site, usually at homeless shelters concentrating on vulnerable populations, shifted to the Red Cross shelter that housed 12,000 evacuees where I would spend 2 days a week with junior nursing students contributing to the relief efforts. I spent many hours helping evacuees obtain prescription medications, contact family members, and providing organizational assistance to the Red Cross nurses in charge. Delivering direct care in this shelter environment made sense to me; here, I knew that our contributions were valued. The learning opportunities were unlike any I had ever experienced, and the students embraced the chance to contribute to the relief efforts in a professional capacity.

Now, I had to enter a classroom to teach the 2-hour elective course. After our emergency response efforts in the shelter, the classroom seemed a surreal environment. How could we go on with a normal class, with business as usual? I anticipated that many of the students were also immersed in the recovery efforts involving their own families or cities nearby. However, they were students, not evacuees. Although we were in a state of emergency and students were affected by the disaster, I was obligated to maintain academic integrity. Before this disaster, senior faculty sometimes reminded me that I am the students' teacher, not their nurse. A "nursectomy" did not seem possible in my case. I have yet to find a way to remove me as nurse from me as teacher. Now I would have to be flexible, assess the situation, and proceed in some manner that addressed course content while taking care of the students.

This was my first semester to teach our new elective course called "Complementary and Integrative Therapies in Health Care." Nineteen students, freshman to seniors, were due to have their second lecture 3 days after Katrina hit. On the lecture schedule was an overview of the concepts integral to the course and the state board's declaratory statement related to Holistic Nursing Practice and Complementary Therapies. The reading assignment, located at the State Board of Nursing Web site, was not accessible because the power had been interrupted to the New Orleans office. The Web site would not be accessible for several months. Many Web-based resources I had come to rely on were disrupted and/or no longer available. Later in the semester, I would learn that frequent disruption of resources that we had come to rely on would become the "new normal."

A retooling of the course content was required. Given the state of emergency and the huge influx of evacuees into our homes, hospitals, and hearts, I knew this would not be a routine semester. The new normal now included a continual awareness of life interrupted: unreliable postal service, phones that do not work, absence of the usual grocery items, and the lives of our relatives east and west of us chronicled on national television weekly (Rose, 2006). I seized the opportunity to talk about trauma, PTSD, and how guided imagery works as a self-soothing tool to evoke a relaxation response (Naparstek, 2004). Although I had originally intended for the class to have interactive features later in the semester, now was the ideal time to become interactive. Therefore, I selected a guided imagery CD about 30 minutes in length designed to enhance performance of any kind, as this seemed appropriate for improving disaster nursing performance (Naparstek & Kohn, 2001).

I opened the class by describing the range of needs I had witnessed in the last 48 hours among the evacuees in the shelter and acknowledged that they, the students, had needs as a result of the disaster. I shared a short version of my own family's concerns, the most pressing of which was locating a developmentally delayed relative who had been sent to the Superdome. He had not been heard from, we could not reach him. We knew the people at the Superdome were being confined to that location as first responders focused on lifesaving rescue, and there was no way to enter a city under lock-down with mandatory evacuations underway. I was at that time and will forever be grateful for the presence of my sister and brother-in-law. They, along with my husband, allowed me to dedicate considerable time in the shelter after class, where I was most useful. Not to mention, I had hoped to be privileged to "inside information" about Superdome evacuations, but the information was sparse and often unreliable.

Today's class, I informed them, would allow students to listen to the CD and to share their own stories. I played the guided imagery CD that evoked calm and invited listeners to see themselves on a screen in their minds' eye performing some activity (Naparstek & Kohn, 2001). The voice guided listeners to breathe deeply and imagine a safe location. Evoking images that are pleasant and nourishing to the senses, an awareness of being surrounded by a cushion of light and being supported in taking action, it provided a concentrated moment of deep relaxation and a renewed sense of confidence (Naparstek & Kohn, 2001). The music contributed to an uplifted feeling and a lightness of being. Afterward, students shared in quiet tones how listening to the CD made them feel calm and instilled a sense of hope and recognition that they were in the right profession. I spoke about the simplicity of taking a deep breath as an intervention for relieving stress. Students were then invited to talk about their families, their experiences, and their concerns. After each story, we would all take a deep breath together.

Sixteen of the 19 students had hurricane-related stories to tell. The family members who were on their couches and in the living rooms of their small, student apartments often brought pets, elders, and small children with them with differing degrees of coping capacities. Many expressed anxiety over their situations. Some were moved to tears by the reports of their fellow students; others were barely able to speak because of their fears for the safety of loved ones whose whereabouts were still unknown. So, it was that we, joined together for fewer than 14 days with a common interest in nursing, spoke about our families, stressors, and fears with considerable authenticity. Entries in weekly journals offer a sense of the reflections shared during that class:

> This is a crazy week. My life has been a mess. Hurricane Katrina hit land Monday and things have been in chaos ever since. My sister and her two disabled kids have come to stay with us. It is hard for me because I have three children of my own. She has been very upset because she lost all of her belongings from the flooding.
>
> We have 12 people in this small 2 bedroom apartment. I feel like I can't even hear myself think. I am worried about my dad and [name]. I know mom is fine.... She had to stay at the hospital. I can't get in touch with dad and my phone isn't working properly. Okay. Deep breath! .... Devastating news about New Orleans... Pray, pray, pray for all of those affected.

Careful not to overwhelm them with too much information when I saw that glassy-eyed, "deer in the headlights" look in students' eyes, I explained PTSD in the briefest of terms—that observing trauma, just as experiencing trauma, could put them at risk. Even watching the images of the aftermath of this hurricane on television was a potential trigger. I told them that nurses were looked on as resource people and were required to be on duty during disasters. People would look to them for strength and information, even though they are only students. Expected to respond to emergencies with clear heads and open hearts and to provide leadership with compassion, they would not have the luxury of falling apart in the face of such immense needs. Therefore, they were obligated to care for themselves, to know when to draw boundaries, and to retreat for self-care needs so that they could continue to be of service. After cautioning the students against watching too much television, I challenged them to find a role that fit their level of skill and desire to contribute. Because giving back to those less fortunate is also a potentially healing tool for the effects of trauma (Naparstek, 2004), I invited them to join me on weekends in the shelter and urged them to take care of themselves.

After this week's class, student journals revealed how the shift from didactic to interactive impacted them:

> Today's class was very touching and laid back. A natural disaster has rocked our state and many lives have changed because of it. Mrs. L. went around the room and had students, who were affected by the hurricane, talk about their feelings and thoughts. She even expressed some of her information, tales and emotions; I was touched by it all.
>
> We had our second class today and discussed what has been happening over the past week. I tried to stay composed but started crying when I was talking about my family and how I have not heard from Pop yet.
>
> [My husband] told me a long time ago what could happen if N.O. was hit by a major hurricane and what is going on right now is how I imagined it!⊗ Unbelievable! Class was emotional. To hear stories of classmates and given the opportunity to de-compartmentalize was wonderful. Keep praying! I feel somewhat selfish because I am saddened that the city I adore is gone, the beautiful place where my husband proposed to me is no longer. So sad!

Other students' entries indicated their appreciation of the benefits of guided imagery:

> I missed the first half of the class but I came in to listen to a "guided imagery" CD. The CD was very calming and relaxing and before I realized it I was sleeping but not soundly. I think you chose a great day and time to share guided imagery with the class because I believe that everyone is affected in one way or another by the destruction of Hurricane Katrina. Just listening to the woman's voice on the CD helped me to get in contact with my inner self. After speaking to you after, I felt it relieved and I went on to work with a sense of hope in my heart. I began to do different things with my family instead of dwelling in front of the news staring at the horrific, but reality scenes on CNN news.
>
> After all had been said we were able to escape from reality with a guided imagery CD. I have never done that before and I am not quite sure if I did it right, but it was a great experience.
>
> We did a guided mediation today and I have not felt that relaxed since all this stuff started with Katrina.

> I was very amazed at how relaxed and good this 30 minute period made me feel. ... I was shocked at how relaxing and real it felt. At one point the woman said to feel someone touching you on your chest and feel the tingling warmth throughout your body, and to my surprise I felt it. It was really cool and moving. The rest of the class we were talking about Hurricane Katrina which I find very depressing so this imagery CD was an awesome escape.

We had just begun to discover the "new normal" when Hurricane Rita formed in the Gulf and headed our way. Although some just boarded up windows and hunkered down because there were not many places left to go, this time we would be the evacuees. After Hurricane Rita, some students returned to find their homes inundated with water from the storm surge. Life was interrupted again. But now, this group of 19 students had new skills in coping and a support group that met each Thursday. It was called class, and I was the nurse/educator guiding them toward different choices as we learned about other pathways to health. One student's final entry into her journal may say it best:

> I really did not regard this as a class in the sense of being in school but more of a spiritual journey for me. Each time I was in the room where class was held, I felt as if I was in a place similar to a "retreat." I can't think of another word, but that is what it felt like. I didn't feel like I was being instructed but guided in a way.

This class, conducted in this state of emergency, was modified to link course content with the primary concerns of students living through the aftermath of Hurricane Katrina. As a teacher, I was able to maintain academic integrity; as a nurse, I helped these students to manage the stress of the now while anticipating the needs for the future.

Students' Stories: The ABCs of Their Reflections

Because we (S. C. P. and A. L. S.) have studied the perceived stress level of students for a number of years, students' stress was clearly evident to us in both classroom and clinical settings after the two hurricanes. We noticed that students wanted to tell us about their experiences and feelings. It seemed very important to them to share stories about personal losses, sheltering family and friends, and being evacuees themselves. Our study of life event stressors among freshman nursing students revealed that students experienced high levels of stress in the best of times (Patel, Sudduth, & Jakopac, 2005).

This was surely not the best of times. It was late November when we regained our own equilibrium and realized the importance of exploring students' stress levels in the aftermath of these major life events. If it took us as faculty 3 months following the hurricanes to regain our balance, we wanted to find out how our students were managing their stressors following the same disasters. We believed we would get the most revealing responses if we asked the students to share while stories were still fresh in their minds before they went home for the holidays to debrief. So, we quickly submitted a research proposal that was approved by the university's Institutional Review Board. This section describes how our interest in student stress translated into a reflective question that yielded rich information about how Hurricanes Katrina and Rita affected the nursing students at the University of Louisiana at Lafayette.

As Jill Laroussini pointed out, both students and faculty returned to the classroom feeling stressed and overwhelmed. Students met the challenges of coming to class and going to clinical experiences while experiencing turmoil in their personal lives. At the end of the semester, students in the College of Nursing were given the opportunity to respond in writing to the question, "Tell us about your experiences or feelings about Hurricanes Katrina and Rita." Sixty-two students volunteered to share their personal stories about their experiences and feelings. In analyzing their stories, we developed an A–B–C formula to organize students' responses. All responses concerning school-related matters were categorized as "A" for academics. Psychological and physical symptoms were filed under "B" for behaviors. Strategies used to deal with hurricane stress were considered "C" for coping.

A for Academics

Slightly more than one-third of the students reported having problems with their academic performance. Many found their academic performance sliding. In fact, two students decided to transfer out because of poor academic performance:

> The hurricane put lots of unwanted stress on the semester prior to clinicals. I'm not happy things turned out this way. It has hurt my grades this semester

but everyone has to deal with it. My GPA dropped a whole point this semester and I'm taking less hours than last semester. (21-year-old male whose family lost their home.)

Due to the hurricanes, I personally felt that I got off to an extremely slow start this semester. At many times I just felt that I was behind and just couldn't quite seem to get caught up. (20-year-old female whose family lost their home.)

The hurricanes have impacted my life somewhat. It's not just family issues but mostly school. School was so messed up from the hurricanes and has put major stress on my shoulders. Everything is happening at once and it's hard to handle. This semester has been very difficult for me unlike the other semesters that weren't so bad. (20-year-old female who had no personal losses.)

B for Behaviors

Behaviors reported by the respondents included both physical and psychological symptoms. Interestingly, only 1 of the 62 students reported physical symptoms of stress:

> I lost both my grandparents due to pneumonia due to evacuating and having decreased immune systems. I now have gastritis and GERD. I am seeing the therapist/taking medication. I lost 10 pounds this semester. (22-year-old female whose family lost their home and sheltered 20 people for 3 weeks.)

The behaviors most frequently reported were psychological. Feelings that repeated themselves in many students' responses included powerlessness, helplessness, disbelief, shock, numbness, guilt, fear, being overwhelmed, anger, worry, and difficulty concentrating. Many shared their grief about the loss of their homes, belongings, and even deaths of family and friends:

> I often felt powerless. I had no control. It took a toll on school performance and my self esteem. I feel I should have done better. (24-year-old female who lost personal and family home and sheltered 2 people for 1 week.)
>
> My seven year old daughter's school was flooded. It took almost a month for them to be placed in another school but they only go on alternative schedule. Monday, Wednesday, Friday one week and second week is Tuesday, Thursday, Saturday. My father has dementia and my mother works so I have to rely on day care. I even had to bring her to school two days because there just wasn't anyone to leave her with. So I sleep about 2 hours a night and pray I will survive the semester. So I can become a nurse while I worry about money and the trauma this is causing my child. So it's a little stressful.

(40-year-old female who experienced personal loss, her family home, and resided in a shelter for 3 days.)

C for Coping

Students' coping behaviors included descriptions of adaptive and maladaptive strategies. The adaptive coping strategies most frequently reported were praying, expressing empathy for others' situations, volunteering, seeking counseling, and expressing gratitude for the good things in life that remained.

> My family experienced a great deal of loss during the hurricane. I never thought at the age of 20 I would have a family of four living with me. The most important thing that I learned was that prayer was the most important medicine and stress, heartache, and disappointments can be given up to God. (20-year-old student.)
>
> Volunteering helped, but at the same time made me more upset to hear and deal with the things that many of the people went through. (25-year-old male without loss of property or family.)
>
> It was a difficult time but when you see how much more difficult other people have it, you feel blessed. (22-year-old whose family home was destroyed.)

With these stories, students shared their lived experience of a natural disaster that is considered by many to be one of the worst in the nation's history in land mass affected, deaths, and personal property destruction. It is amazing to us that the students were so resilient and kept on going and meeting the demands of the academic curriculum despite their personal losses and grief. Several students at the end of their stories thanked us for the opportunity to express their feelings and to tell us how they were coping. Overall, these students surprised themselves with how well they seem to be doing academically, behaviorally, and implementing positive coping strategies in the face of personal tragedy.

It was good news to us to learn that our students seemed to be holding their own early in the process of recovery. Because we know that students' early responses may not be a clear indication of adaptive coping, during spring semester 2006, we will be on the look out for indications of PTSD effects in students related to the hurricanes. We plan to query the students before they leave for summer break to study their reflections 9 months after the hurricanes.

Faculty Stories: The Eye of the Storm

Within the center of any hurricane lies the eye of the storm, a place of calm where the winds die down and sun beams through. Years of cooperation and collaboration in a trusting environment no doubt contributed to our ability as a faculty group to act as a peaceful presence as chaos swhirled around us. In the College of Nursing and across campus, we worked to make school as normal as possible and encouraged students to stay focused on their studies. This proved to be a challenge because many of us were dealing with our own personal disasters. In many ways, we were no different from the students. Our homes had become temporary refuges for extended periods of time as our evacuee guests wondered if their homes were underwater and would ever be habitable again. In this section, Gwen Leigh shares stories of how she and her faculty colleagues served as role models who helped students to cope while dealing with their own hurricane-related challenges.

As faculty, we often found ourselves counting our blessings because we all knew someone who had family members missing, or injured, or worse. Gwen's (my) retired in-laws lost what they had worked years for, a camp on the Mississippi Gulf Coast and a 30-foot sailboat. As a part-time nursing staff member, 3 days after Katrina, I was called in to assist when my local hospital became the staging area for the evacuation of the Tulane Medical Center in New Orleans. Tulane employees, families, and even pets were air-lifted by helicopter from the roof of the downtown medical center to buses that brought them 2 hours west to our hospital. No one was allowed to evacuate with shoes as the potential for contamination was too great. I worked late into the night helping to get these evacuees out of contaminated clothing and into showers—their first in 3 days. After the showers, I provided clean clothes, stuffed animals for the children, and a compassionate ear while listening to many stories of care and sacrifice.

Nurses told me how the food supplies had become so seriously depleted that they ate small portions of junk food for 2 days so their patients had more to eat. They had to ration drinking water for both staff and patients. The toilets had not worked since the levees broke. There were no clean linens and the electricity was out. Generators had stopped worked so the only source of illumination when caring for patients day and night came from small flashlights. One said, "If I never see a flashlight again, it will be too soon." In the sweltering heat, patients had to be evacuated through dark stairwells once again using flashlights to see where they were going. Many expressed regret at having to leave the hospital knowing that nursing staff and patients across the street at Charity Hospital were still waiting to be evacuated. Some told me how they walked through the high flood waters to bring their remaining drinking water, food and supplies to Charity Hospital after their patients had been evacuated.

In sharing such stories with others at the College of Nursing, I realized how much better I felt afterwards. Because my faculty colleagues had their own stories to tell, I decided to collect them. Not only to keep a record of these life-altering events, but also to allow them to unburden themselves. Expressions of gratitude were common during this stressful time:

> For Hurricane Katrina, I had my daughter, son-in-law and grandchild living with us for five weeks. For three of those weeks they did not know if they had a house and one of their cars to return to. My son-in-law knew for certain that his mother's house was completely under water! Both my daughter and son-in-law are registered nurses and the hospital they worked in was destroyed and they did not where they would find jobs. When Hurricane Rita hit, my brother and his wife came to stay and that was an overlap with our other evacuees for a week. My home went from two adults and one cat to six adults, an infant, five cats and one dog. For three days my brother did not know if he had a home or business to return to. But we were all together and all alive. Many people could not say that.

Many of my faculty colleagues felt less helpless when they answered the call for nurses at the evacuation centers. Despite the tense situation on campus, in spite of the additional work of adjusting their courses, and with households full of "guests," many dealt with their stress by volunteering. One such faculty volunteer even found a "lost" relative in the process:

> I was in an automobile accident before Katrina and had a cervical injury. I was not feeling well during this time and had reservations about volunteering at the shelter. However, I was compelled to do some type of volunteer work to help out. The outpouring of goodness in our community was overwhelming to me. I elected to volunteer at the emergency room at a local hospital. I was able to triage patients in from New Orleans. God is good! One of the patients I happened to triage was my aunt from New Orleans, who had a gastrointestinal bleed from the stress of the storm. She stayed in the hospital for three days and then came home with me. Volunteering helped me adapt to the stress, even if it was just for an eight hour shift. After we got my family placed we heard from another aunt and my uncle. They were evacuated to

a local nursing home. My uncle was in a nursing home in New Orleans and my aunt accompanied him when they evacuated. He died at the local nursing home after being evacuated from New Orleans. My aunt called me during the night. She could not say enough good things about the nurses who cared for my uncle. Her dilemma was where to send his body. He had wanted it donated to Tulane Medical School in New Orleans, however there was no Tulane. This aunt came and stayed with me, along with her daughter, who flew in from Chicago until after the service. Again, this community was awesome to my family, from the priest who said the funeral to friends who supported not only our family, but now my extended family who now was in Lafayette. I am forever grateful for this wonderful community I live in.

Although not all faculty members were personally impacted, every faculty member felt the effect of Hurricane Katrina, as educators were called on to be flexible in ways they never anticipated. Instead of presenting lectures, many had to place notes and PowerPoint presentations on BlackBoard for students to read on their own. Lectures had to be consolidated. Portions of courses were suddenly self-study, and examinations had to be postponed, some more than once. BlackBoard became the most reliable way to communicate with students.

> As course coordinator, I had many issues to deal with. Students were stranded in other states and one of my students was activated by the National Guard as a result of Katrina. Lectures were either rescheduled or placed on BlackBoard, with students instructed to thoroughly read this content in their textbooks.

Faculty expressed some of the same feelings as the students about being displaced and looking for a normal life:

> I guess overall, the biggest effect on me was a feeling of uncertainty about life in general and the realization that none of us are in control of the things that we take for granted such as shelter, finances, safety, and family. Close friends experienced loss of their homes, and my family prayed a lot for those not as fortunate as we were. Looking ahead was difficult, and we felt compelled to watch tragic situations and events on TV, sometimes for hours on end. Now, people are actively working to rebuild what was lost, and a sense of normalcy is returning. But we do somewhat dread another hurricane season, and pray that we are spared for many more years.

As everyone on the coast was still trying to comprehend the impact of Hurricane Katrina, our world was again turned upside down as Hurricane Rita took aim at Louisiana. I will share my own observations of the challenges faced by our faculty group before and after this second hurricane. It was Thursday morning, and I was working in the simulation laboratory with the students. Our department head interrupted the students to announce that all students and personnel living in Vermillion, Iberia, and St. Martin parishes were excused from all classes immediately. A mandatory evacuation had just been called for these regions south and southwest of the university. Another major hurricane was heading our way! Students were instructed to go home, pack what they could, and to evacuate to at least 100 miles north of Lafayette. Just a couple of hours later, the department head again interrupted with the news that the entire university was closing in 1 hour and would be closed until further notice. Faculty were instructed to back up anything important on their office computers on discs. We were to take those discs and anything else we might need to conduct our courses from a remote location. In addition, it was recommended that we pick everything up off the floor and take anything valuable in our offices.

Nobody expected to have to apply the lessons learned from Hurricane Katrina so soon. We knew not to depend solely on our cell phones because, following Katrina, the Internet proved to be the most reliable form of communication. Before leaving, both the dean and the department head updated all faculty members' personal cell phone numbers, e-mail addresses, and the landline phone numbers in the event that we were evacuated, we could be contacted. Anticipating probable power outages that would disable the university computer server for an indeterminate length of time, we exchanged personal e-mail addresses.

With all of the hotels, shelters, and even campgrounds in Louisiana and the nearby states filled above capacity with Hurricane Katrina evacuees, our most pressing question became where could those running from Hurricane Rita go? Without knowing the answer, we left wishing everyone well and telling each other to stay safe. Once again, our city and university were spared major damage, although we did experience widespread power outages. The areas just south and west of us were not as fortunate, and we began to accept evacuees from those regions into our shelters. Despite devastating destruction just 17 miles south of the university, we reopened the following Tuesday.

That weekend, our dean and department head flew to Baltimore to accept the National League for Nursing's 2005 Center of Excellence in Nursing Education™ award for "Creating Environments That Promote Ongoing Faculty Development." As it turned out, it was the same "empowerment culture" that brought our College of Nursing recognition as a National League for Nursing Center of Excellence that sustained faculty and students with a sense of community as strong as our commitment to excellence. Commencement is a perfect example. Graduation exercises were usually held at the Cajun Dome and the adjoining Conference Center. Less than 15 business days before the event, the university was notified that the Cajun Dome would not be available. Plans to move the commencement exercises to smaller venues across campus resulted in a domino effect of consequences that included restricting students to a set number of guests. New invitations were actually printed and mailed to the graduating seniors before commencement.

Despite all of the problems we faced, our College of Nursing was one of the few schools of nursing along the Louisiana and Mississippi Gulf Coast to graduate on time. At the end of the semester luncheon celebration, our department head told us that she believed we were all suffering from PTSD. She encouraged us to make a special effort to be with family and enjoy our holidays during Christmas break.

Lessons Learned: Tips for Nurse Educators Facing Disasters

In the aftermath of these two hurricanes, the resourcefulness of our faculty group was proportionate to the stressors. This disaster actually gifted us with the challenge of turning obstacles into opportunities. Jill Laroussini learned that balancing flexibility with maintaining academic commitments inspired her to actively engage students in implementing guided visulization as a self-care tool, thereby addressing their primary concerns in the aftermath of these natural disasters. *Jill's Tip*: Seize the moment to teach your students positive coping strategies, ranging from simply focusing on the breath to more complex self-care interventions.

Following any major disaster, Sudha Patel and Ardith Sudduth knew that faculty and students will experience a period of grief and loss. They learned that faculty members are ideally positioned to carefully listen to students, to identify needs, and to be vigilant in observing the effects of stress immediately after a disaster and in the semesters to follow. *Sudha and Ardith's Tip*: Trust yourself to be responsive to students' stress because the usual resources from the university and community may become unavailable under disaster conditions.

From her own experience, Gwen learned the cathartic and therapeutic effect of telling her story to faculty colleagues. Besides caring for students in the midst of a disaster, faculty must take the time to care for themselves. *Gwen's Tip*: To be a true role model to your students, share your stories with your faculty colleagues, volunteer to help with relief efforts, and take time for yourself to rest and recharge.

Conclusion

This chapter deals with the healing power of stories. These stories detail the experiences of faculty and students in the aftermath of the two hurricanes that hit the Louisiana coast in 2005; and they also describe how cathartic it was to share these stories—whether we told them or wrote them down - as we faced the catastrophic and the unfathomable. There are so many stories to share from this experience, stories of resolve and flexibility, resourcefulness, and strength. We have learned that, in times of crisis, everyone's story is important to tell. It was how we processed our experiences and came to understand our strengths, accept our shortcomings, and sift out the important stuff from all the rest. This is why dancing with hurricanes, rather than struggling against them, helped us to regain our balance in the new normal. We are grateful for this opportunity to share our stories with you. We hope you will never have to experience a disaster like ours. Should you ever, remember what we learned: Sharing stories is as much a part of coping as it is a part of creating a community among faculty and students that contributes to everyone's healing.

REFERENCES

Department of Homeland Security. (2005). *Hurricane Katrina: Overview*. Retrieved February 10, 2006, from http://www.dhs.gov/interweb/assetlibrary/katrina.htm

Naparstek, B. (2004) *Invisible heroes: Survivors of trauma and how they heal.* New York: Bantam Dell.

Naparstek, B., & Kohn, S. M. (2001). *A meditation to help you improve self-confidence and reach peak performance.* [CD-ROM]. Ohio: Health Journeys.

Patel, S., Sudduth, A., & Jakopac, K. (2005, July). Self-reported life stressors among students in their first nursing course [Abstract]. *Proceedings of the 16th International Nursing Research Congress Sigma Theta Tau International.* (Proceedings made available in the Virginia Henderson Sigma Theta Tau Library.)

Rose, C. (2006, January 24). Our lives have become must see TV. *The Times Picayune.* Retrieved January 26, 2006, from http://www.nola.com

Chapter 8

The Ultimate Challenge: Three Situations Call American Nurses to Think and Act Globally

Ruth Neese, Gene Majka, and Geneiva G. Tennant

N urse educators in the United States face many challenges: a serious nursing shortage putting pressure on educators to produce more nurses, more qualified students seeking entry into nursing programs than faculty available to teach them, a lack of nursing faculty to replace retirees, and inconsistent health literacy in clients and students. As doctoral students in South Florida, we were surprised to learn that nurse educators in the United States are not alone in their struggles to educate sufficient numbers of nurses prepared to deal with a diverse population of students and clients. Coping with the day-to-day demands inherent in the amazing cultural diversity of students in South Florida, we never looked beyond state borders for national or international influences on nursing education. Caught up in the immediacy of meeting multiple challenges, it is easy to miss the local implications of three global challenges: (1) the brain drain of educated professionals migrating from less developed countries (LDCs) to more developed countries (MDCs), (2) the shortage of nursing faculty, and (3) the relationship of literacy and nursing students.

How will these three situations affect American nurse educators? Attracting nurses away from their countries may serve us in the short

This chapter was accepted on April 10, 2006.

term; but, over time, this drain undermines social justice and violates the ethical principle of beneficence, thereby inhibiting efforts at international cooperation among nurse educators. This will make addressing the global nursing faculty shortage at the international level difficult if not impossible. Add the global nurse educator shortage to lower literacy levels and you have a situation where there are fewer qualified nurse educators to prepare less-well qualified students to care for greater numbers of sicker patients. Only a global community of nurse educators can hope to address these issues by acting locally and thinking globally.

This chapter describes the global nature of these three challenges for nursing education, explains how American educators are affected by these challenges, and offers local strategies these educators can use to meet these global challenges. Beyond raising the consciousness of U.S. nurse educators about how these three global situations impinge on their professional lives, this chapter offers suggestions for local action, as well as participation in global nursing education forums like the National League for Nursing and the International Council of Nurses.

Global Nature of Brain Drain

Although the term "brain drain" has been used in science and technology literature since the 1960s, it did not appear in nursing literature until 1990 (Ortin, 1990). Brain drain is defined in *Merriam-Webster's Collegiate Dictionary* as, "the departure of educated or professional people from one country, economic sector, or field to another usually for better pay or living conditions" (Mish, 2001, p. 138). As educated professionals, nurses are "voting with their feet" and leaving LDCs in large numbers. Thus, brain drain depletes poorer countries of nurses and widens the gap in health inequities worldwide (Pang, Lansang, & Haines, 2002). The purpose of this section is to briefly describe the global nature of brain drain, the effects of this drain on American nurse educators, and local strategies educators can use to meet this challenge.

Ten years after Dr. Francois Duvalier came to power in Haiti, the one and only state medical school graduated 264 physicians; all but three left the country (Farmer, 1999). This drain also occurs with nurses in many developed and LDCs. The International Monetary Fund ranks Iran as having the highest rate (approximately 200,000 professionals per year) of brain drain in the world (Dehghanpisheh, 2004). Africa, India, Pakistan, and the Philippines are other sources of intellectual labor for developed countries (Llana, 2006).

There are many factors driving the brain drain of nurses from LDCs, some personal and some societal. Personal reasons for immigrating include higher wages, promotion opportunities, guaranteed work, professional opportunities unavailable at home, and improved living conditions ("National Strategies," 2004). Societal factors spurring nurse immigration are poor working conditions, inadequate facilities, limited career structure, threats to personal safety from violence or endemic infections, persecution of intellectuals, political repression, and discrimination (Kingma, 2001; Pang et al., 2002).

Increased income is a major stimulus for the movement of health care professionals to MDCs, and nurses are no exception. Lured by higher wages, the immigration of foreign nurses to the United States has tripled since 2004 (Llana, 2006). Nurses who come to the United States to work use technologically advanced equipment, adopt evidence-based models of practice, enhance their economic potential, and expand educational opportunities for their children (Meleis, 2003). When these nurses do not return home, LDCs do not benefit from their expanded knowledge base.

More developed countries are not immune to brain drain; Europe contributes to and suffers from brain drain. Western Europe recruits nurses from African nations and loses researchers to the United States. About 50% of Europeans completing their PhDs in the United States remain here for long periods after completion, and many stay permanently (Bosch, 2003). This applies to nurse educators as well.

Effects of Brain Drain on American Nurse Educators

Why should American nurse educators care about brain drain? On the surface, it appears to be a win-win situation. Nurses from LDCs fill vacant educator positions in the United States, and these immigrant educators get higher wages and better living conditions for themselves and their families. The appearance of win-win is an illusion. Brain drain marks a potentially serious barrier to economic growth, development, poverty reduction, and improving health care in developing countries. Academics and others are important in developing countries given their role in research, innovation, teaching, and training (Shanahan, 2005). These "others" include nurse educators. Nursing education does not exist solely to provide students with a skill set available to the highest bidder; nursing education exists to teach providers how to improve the health of their communities equitably.

Every skilled nurse who migrates leaves thousands of poor without health care. When a nurse educator immigrates, this effect is compounded by the loss of someone who can teach others to fill the widening gaps in health care. Our nursing codes of ethics (American Nurses Association, 2001; International Council of Nurses, 2000) demand attention to social justice and the ethical principle of beneficence. Siphoning skilled nurses from LDCs violates these principles by leaving already vulnerable populations at higher risk of ill health and crippling the educational infrastructure needed to meet the health needs of these countries. Local strategies that U.S. educators can use to address the brain drain problem must emphasize equity and beneficence.

Local Strategies for Nurse Educators in Addressing Brain Drain

There is no one single solution to the brain drain problem. Proposed solutions have to be two-fold. First, LDCs must reduce the factors that prompt nurse educators to immigrate and find a means to retain their professionals within their boundaries. Second, MDCs must reduce excessive recruiting and foster the return of educators to their home countries.

Strategy 1: Curbing the Need to Recruit From Less Developed Countries

Retaining nurse educators in their current positions and developing new educators are obvious solutions that have received much attention in the literature. Another strategy involves working with LDCs to develop a world-class nursing education forum. This program would allow participating countries to share the expertise of nurse educators, but keep their own personnel resources. In countries that have the infrastructure, Web-based synchronous and asynchronous discussion could support such a forum. U.S. nurse educators can participate in this strategy by developing Web-based forums and supporting global nursing organizations' efforts to mitigate immigration and cultivate "home-grown" nurse educators. The International Council of Nurses is working to implement this type of program.

Strategy 2: Using Fair Recruiting Practices

The United Kingdom National Health Services developed international recruitment protocols that prohibit recruiting from countries that are hemorrhaging health care personnel, educators included (Shanahan, 2005). Nurse educators in the United States can develop similar protocols through national nursing organizations. These protocols can also call for the compensation of poor countries for the loss of skilled nurse educators as reimbursement for the cost of replacement. Schools and universities that recruit nurse educators from LDCs could offer only short-term contracts to encourage these educators to return home (Buchan, 2001). Finally, U.S. nurse educators can foster the return of immigrants to their home countries by supporting "return of talent" programs sponsored by international nursing organizations.

Global Nature of the Nursing Faculty Shortage

The shift of highly educated nurses from LDCs to MDCs through brain drain is one factor contributing to the global nursing faculty shortage. Other contributing factors vary based on the country or global region being discussed. A global nursing faculty shortage is impairing the education of nurses and interfering with the development of nursing knowledge. In the United States, nursing faculty are well acquainted with high vacancy rates in teaching positions. Globally, the faculty shortage must be inferred from an absolute lack of practicing nurses. The International Council of Nurses reports ratios of 71 nurses per 100,000 population in Africa and 59 nurses per 100,000 population in Southeast Asia (Buchan & Calman, 2004). Regional variations within countries indicate even more severe shortages, especially in sub-Saharan Africa (Buchan & Calman, 2004). A combination of different mechanisms is driving this shortage.

The mechanisms underlying the nursing faculty shortage vary by global region. Thoroughly analyzed and reported in the nursing literature, the mechanisms in North America and much of Europe are an aging workforce, institutional budgetary constraints, declining graduate enrollments, academic role demands, and increasing financial incentives to remain in clinical practice (AACN, 2003; Berlin & Sechrist, 2002; Brendtro & Hegge, 2000; DeYoung, Bliss, & Tracy, 2002; Emerson & Records, 2005).

Different mechanisms contribute to the nursing faculty shortage in Latin America, Asia, Africa, and the Near East. Many of the countries in these regions lack graduate schools of nursing due to inadequate economic and infrastructure resources, hindering the education and development of nursing faculty (Anders & Kunaviktikul, 1999; Buchan & Calman, 2004; Jarrett, Hummel & Whitney, 2005; Ketefian, Daly, Chang, & Srisuphan, 2005; Sigma Theta Tau International, 2003). Another common problem is the use of physicians and other nonnursing personnel as educators and administrators in schools of nursing (International Council of Nurses, 2004; Jarrett et al., 2005; Ketefian et al., 2005; Sigma Theta Tau International, 2003). This impedes nursing knowledge development and role definition in the affected countries. Finally, many of the countries in these regions display pronounced gender inequality with its accompanying structural violence, which is pervasive institutionalized discrimination and denial of personhood to women that limits women's roles and potential (Buchan & Calman, 2004; Farmer, 2005; Lopez-Claros & Zahidi, 2006). Because nurses are predominantly female, structural violence denies nurses the opportunity for advanced education, limits their scope of practice, impedes their ability to conduct research, and traps many in resource-poor practice settings and schools (Buchan & Calman, 2004; Girot & Enders, 2004; Jarrett et al., 2005; Sigma Theta Tau International, 2003). Lack of graduate education, nonnurse educators, and gender inequality combine to create a nursing faculty shortage in these regions.

Effect of Global Faculty Shortage on American Nurse Educators

Why should a global nursing faculty shortage concern American nurse educators? A lack of qualified nursing faculty means many immigrating nurses may not meet U.S. standards for nursing practice. Ill-prepared nurses who immigrate from LDCs increase demands for refresher classes, adding burdens to nurse educators' already packed schedules. Actively recruiting faculty from other countries may fill vacancies in the short term, but can decimate resource-poor nursing schools in LDCs by luring away already scarce educators. Fewer educators mean more ill-prepared students, setting up a vicious cycle and perpetuating images of nurses as undereducated and subservient. Draining educators to the West does not foster international goodwill, interfering with faculty exchange programs and the development of an internationally standardized nursing curriculum. Nursing knowledge development is impeded when there are too few doctorally prepared nurses available to conduct nursing research and role model nursing as an intellectual enterprise (Emerson & Records, 2005; Hinshaw, 2001; McGivern, 2003). Taken together, these issues suggest the need for solutions to the nursing faculty shortage. Because there are a variety of factors fueling the shortage, a variety of local actions will be needed to meet this global challenge.

Local Strategies for Nurse Educators to Address the Global Faculty Shortage

Many strategies for solving the nursing faculty shortage have been proposed. The primary solution offered for all countries has been the recruitment of younger undergraduate students to speed through accelerated doctoral programs into faculty positions (AACN, 2003; Berlin & Sechrist, 2002; Buchan & Calman, 2004; DeYoung, Bliss, & Tracy, 2002; Emerson & Records, 2005; Hinshaw, 2001; McGivern, 2003). This position of more, younger, and faster has been offered as the solution to every nursing shortage. Continued fixation on this solution displays ageist bias and ignores demographic data on nursing students and the larger population.

The age of undergraduate and graduate nursing students in MDCs has been rising to 40 and over. This mirrors a global population trend that began appearing by 1990 (Kinsella & Velkoff, 2001). Median age in MDCs and LDCs is predicted to rise above 35 years of age by 2030, with the exception of sub-Saharan Africa (Kinsella & Velkoff, 2001). Most developed nations in North America, Europe, and South America will have median ages at or over 40 by 2030 (Kinsella & Velkoff, 2001). The hoped-for pool of young undergraduates will not be there to solve the faculty shortage. Local strategies must focus on developing nurse educators using the available pool of middle-aged students and forging connections between individuals, institutions, and nations. Four strategies are proposed that address resolution of entry into practice, development of nurse educators, establishment of mutually beneficial partnerships, and creation of research consortiums.

Strategy 1: Resolve Entry Into Practice Issues

Unlike many LDCs, much of the developed world offers multiple ways for students to enter nursing practice. Hospital-based diploma programs, associate degrees from community colleges, and baccalaureate degrees from universities all grant the title of "nurse." This brands nursing as a "confusing, poorly differentiated occupation of menial tasks" (David, 2000, p. 87) and perpetuates class, gender, and socioeconomic biases. Undereducated nurses often fail to recognize their disadvantage and do not aspire to graduate education (David, 2000; Roberts, 2000). Failure to resolve the entry into practice issue will contribute to a continuing decline in graduate enrollment. Nurse educators must collaborate with state boards of nursing and nurses' associations to establish a baccalaureate degree in nursing as the basic educational requirement for nursing practice, which lays the groundwork for graduate education.

Strategy 2: Develop Nurse Educators

Nurses are needed to teach nurses and advance nursing knowledge. Non-nurses who teach nursing in LDCs must be replaced by nurse educators. In many MDCs, the educator role was de-emphasized and the clinician role promoted in graduate education (DeYoung, Bliss, & Tracy, 2002; Hinshaw, 2001; Kelly, 2002). This was done based on the assumption that clinical graduate education prepared one to teach, an assumption proven inaccurate. Nursing graduate students need deliberate preparation as educators, including a mentored teaching practicum (DeYoung, Bliss, & Tracy; Kelly, 2002; National League for Nursing, 2002; Neese, 2003). This need for deliberate preparation applies whether the students are in developed or developing countries.

Nurse educators can implement this strategy by:

1. Promoting the nurse educator role by renewing emphasis on educator preparation and the importance of effective teaching in the preparation of skilled nurses.

2. Resisting ageist bias by recruiting promising undergraduate and graduate students to the educator role *regardless of their age.*
3. Combating sexism that blocks female nurses from faculty positions by partnering in grassroots efforts for gender equity with indigenous feminist organizations like the National Organization for Women, Isis International, Association for Women's Rights in Development, Union Nacional de Mujeres Guatemaltecas (National Union of Guatemalan Women), and the Global Fund for Women.
4. Ensuring availability of flexible master's and PhD programs to meet the needs of middle-aged students.
5. Supporting efforts by indigenous nursing associations and the International Council of Nurses to promote graduate nursing education in developing countries.

Strategy 3: Establish Mutually Beneficial Partnerships

Informal, mutually supportive relationships assist nurse faculty in coping with feelings of isolation, hierarchical power structures, and hostile work environments (Glass, 2001; 2003). Informal and formal supportive relationships help new doctoral graduates negotiate their development into confident nurse-scholars (Heinrich, 2005). Formal mutually beneficial partnerships may be used to foster individual faculty development, facilitate collaboration between disciplines and institutions, and promote the international exchange of nursing education research and knowledge (Heinrich et al., 2003, 2004). These partnerships have negotiated contracts, a timetable for achieving goals, are open to renegotiation, and are based on mutual respect (Heinrich et al., 2003, 2004).

The knowledge development and mutual support obtained through partnerships is reciprocal, empowering, and invigorating (Heinrich et al., 2003, 2004). The use of mutually beneficial partnerships can ease the faculty shortage. Nurse educators can implement this strategy by using partnerships to encourage students to choose nursing education as a career, mentor novice faculty, foster faculty development, and cultivate confidence in scholarly work. These partnerships can also link institutions to facilitate a complementary use of differences when there are gaps in faculty knowledge or expertise. Finally, these partnerships can connect American nurse educators with their peers internationally to facilitate reciprocal knowledge exchange.

Strategy 4: Create Research Consortiums

The major objection voiced to middle-aged nursing faculty was their ab-breviated career path with less time for productive research before retire-ment (AACN, 2003; Berlin & Sechrist, 2002; DeYoung, Bliss, & Tracy, 2002; Emerson & Records, 2005; Hinshaw, 2001; McGivern, 2003). This objection displayed an ageist, androcentric bias that marginalized middle-aged students and educators and privileged individual achieve-ment over collective effort (Bronstein, 2001; Maguire, 2001). Despite this objection, nursing must work with the pool of researchers it has—primarily midlife women. Collaboration, collective effort, and mutual support must be emphasized to perpetuate nursing knowledge devel-opment with this population (Bronstein, 2001; Glass, 2003; Heinrich, 2005; Lesser et al., 2004; Maguire, 2001).

Nurse educators can implement this strategy by developing re-search consortiums that emphasize collective effort on a common re-search thread rather than individual success in obtaining grants. This is not "trickle down" money distributed by tier 1 research institutions to "poorer cousins." These consortiums would be linkages with level power structures, not hierarchies, and could involve individuals, in-stitutions, government offices, nongovernment organizations, or any combination of these entities. Pooling resources would bolster nursing education research (which attracts limited funding), distribute fund-ing more equitably, and complement the relational skills of midlife nurse researchers. Emphasizing the research thread rather than indi-vidual programs would also permit knowledge development to con-tinue, regardless of faculty retirements. Promoting the establishment of these consortiums would tip academic culture (Gladwell, 2002) away from one that favors individual achievement to one that is relational in nature.

Global Influences on Literacy and Nursing Students

A global contributor to ill-prepared students is poor basic education leading to low literacy skills. Being able to read and understand the written word is a vital skill in today's world that affects health and so-cioeconomic status. This section will give an overview of literacy and the effects of illiteracy on students and American educators. Local strategies for dealing with the challenge of illiteracy will be outlined. The United Nations defines illiteracy as the inability to read and write a simple sentence in any language. In the developing world, more than 135 million children between the ages of 7 and 18 have never been to school (Gordon, 2003). Globally, more than 100 million children aged 6–12 are not enrolled in primary school, whereas 137 million young people will begin their adult lives lacking the basic skills of literacy (United Nations Educational, Scientific & Cultural Organization [UNESCO], 2004). The effects of illiteracy can be very far reaching. When a parent cannot read, often their families are caught up in a generational cycle of lack of education, illness, and poverty (World Bank Group, 2001). Illiterate, hungry people in poor health do not aspire to higher education and often immigrate in an attempt to improve their quality of life. This deprives LDCs of human resource potential and transfers the problems caused by illiteracy to MDCs.

Efforts to stem brain drain and foster graduate education for nurses in LDCs will meet limited success if a demographic is ignored—the vast majority of nurses worldwide are female. Unfortunately, gender is linked to another more disappointing statistic caused by structural violence—of the 771 million illiterate adults, two-thirds are women (UNESCO, 2005). Uneducated women doubt their abilities and do not aspire to higher education (Women in Literacy, 2005). Literate women are more confident of their abilities and take better care of their health and that of their families, regardless of where they live (UNESCO, 2005). Children of literate mothers are more likely to read and persist in school (Krashen, 2005).

Low literacy levels greatly affect the readiness of students. The National Survey of America's College Students (Baer, Cook, & Baldi, 2006) reported a strong correlation between requisites of country of birth, personal/parental income, financial dependence, parent's education, years elapsed between high school and entrance into college, and the country in which the students attended high school. Students who graduated from U.S. high schools had higher literacy levels than students who graduated from foreign high schools. Lower family income, parents who did not graduate from high school, and being a member of an ethnic minority all negatively affected literacy. Students enrolled in 2-year colleges had lower literacy levels and professional expectations than those enrolled in 4-year institutions. Having moderate-to-high literacy levels did not correlate with computer literacy, even among licensed professionals

(Wilbright et al., 2006). These global and national influences on literacy definitely affect nurse educators.

Effects of Global Literacy Rates on American Nurse Educators

Why should global literacy rates concern American nurses? Literacy problems hinder overall student success (Baer, Cook, & Baldi, 2006) and have far-reaching implications for nursing's future. Low literacy impacts both the preparedness of prospective nursing students and the likelihood of choosing nursing as a career. Poorly prepared students are at higher risk of failure, and require more time and resources from nurse educators. Students with marginal-to-low literacy skills avoid careers that require high-level reading or math competencies (Baer, Cook, & Baldi, 2006). Foreign students and ethnic minorities in nursing schools are more likely to have low literacy skills, particularly those entering 2-year colleges. Computer literacy demands are now added to basic literacy requirements, and institutional expectations for computer literacy are not being met by graduates (Wilbright et al., 2006). Nurse educators are caught between struggling high-risk students and political pressure to crank out more successful graduates. Ignoring literacy issues in the larger population will contribute to higher numbers of ill-prepared students entering nursing programs. This would increase the need for nursing educators to "weed out" weaker students, thereby ending the dreams of a nursing career for some students. Literacy must be a focus for local action by nurse educators.

Local Strategies for American Nurse Educators to Address Global Literacy Rates

Rapid technological changes, including computer literacy requirements, demand more complex basic literacy competencies for daily living. Literacy campaigns are essential to appropriately prepare future nurses. There are many solutions to this problem, but they all are dependent on a commitment from everyone involved. Four strategies are proposed that focus on the context of literacy needs, policy development, including marginalized populations in literacy campaigns, and emphasizing early childhood development.

Strategy 1: Designing Context-Specific Literacy Initiatives

Literacy campaigns must be grounded in people's everyday realities and normal ways of living. Specific lifestyles and daily schedules should be considered when designing and implementing literacy modules. This would ensure greater participation by those who stand to benefit most. Nursing networks exist in communities with diverse populations. Nursing presence facilitates the collection of first-hand information, with needs analyses and ongoing evaluations of literacy programs through onsite observations. These data can then be used to improve literacy initiatives and shape curricula that are geared to these populations (Nunes & Gaibel, 2002). Literacy campaigns that anticipate and respond to specific groups can foster better-prepared students and positively impact the success of future nursing students.

Strategy 2: Participating in Policy Development

Nurse educators can raise awareness among policy makers about the effects and implications of literacy issues on student populations, such as the potential for failure in educational programs due to inadequate preparation and substandard knowledge base. Increased awareness will help to focus public attention on perspectives and guidelines that govern the development of essential literacy campaigns. Through involvement at local and state levels, nursing has the power to influence and guide the focus of policy initiatives. Local and state nursing associations, with input from its membership, can advise and guide policy development.

Strategy 3: Designing Community Education/Training Initiatives

Many literacy campaigns have failed because they neglected to involve "the voices of the poor" in determining programs that can enhance literacy capability. Including the marginalized in planning these initiatives aids program success. Literacy campaigns at grassroots levels in local churches, synagogues, and meeting places will provide avenues for devising and directing population-specific instruction strategies. Peck, Flower, and Higgins (1995) recommend the use of Freire's (1970) participatory approach in community empowerment strategies.

Members of these communities are required to make suggestions and be actively involved in the development of literacy programs that respond to their needs.

Nurse educators and their students work in many poor and marginalized communities. The development of community-specific literacy initiatives through ongoing class projects will serve to clarify the view of health as a relationship among nurses, clients, and their environments. Health education, which is influenced by issues of literacy, is a major function of nursing. Nutbeam (2000) maintained that health literacy is a key outcome of health education. Linkages to health education in literacy campaigns provide individuals with the capacity to obtain, process, and understand the basic health information and service needed to make appropriate health decisions.

Strategy 4: Emphasizing Early Childhood Development

Frequent book reading by parents to children, which facilitates life-long learning, has been found to impact literacy achievement positively in later years. Maternal book reading and sharing strategies can help in multigenerational literacy development (Calamai, 2000). Nursing, through instructional modules, educates mothers during the perinatal period. Teaching students to include information on the importance of parental book reading in perinatal educational sessions can positively impact literacy development. Nursing students can also reinforce and role model the importance of reading to children during pediatric clinical rotations. Early literacy skills can also be developed through programs like "Reach Out and Read" (2003), which provide books in pediatric primary care settings.

Summary

This chapter discussed the global nature of brain drain, the nursing faculty shortage, literacy, and how these problems affect U.S. nurse educators. Suggestions for action at the local level were made that encourage educator participation in meeting these challenges. To meet the global challenge of brain drain on a local level, U.S. nurse educators must support efforts to end the faculty shortage here and ensure that fair recruiting practices are used when seeking educators from LDCs.

A vigorous recruitment program must be created to bring nurse educators back home to counter the West's lure to leave their home country.
Many international and national nursing organizations are working on
the brain drain problem, and input and support from creative nurse
educators would be welcome.

Four strategies to address the global nursing faculty shortage locally were proposed. First, make a baccalaureate degree in nursing the
minimum academic credential for entry into practice. Second, foster
development of nursing faculty by promoting the role of nurse educator, combating institutional sexism through grassroots activism, recruit
students from all age groups, and work with national and international
nursing organizations to promote graduate nursing education. Third,
develop mutually beneficial partnerships that nurture faculty development and foster collaboration on local, national, and international levels.
Finally, establish research consortiums that complement the relational
strengths of middle-aged nurse researchers by emphasizing collective
effort instead of individual achievement.

Four strategies for nurse educators who want to combat poor literacy and foster better-prepared students in local communities were
shared. These strategies include policy development with programs that
specifically target the poor and marginalized sectors of society with explicit linkages to the influence of literacy on health. Literacy and health
education campaigns must view peoples' ways of living as major considerations and attempt to incorporate local need when devising specific
programs and educational strategies. Nurse educators and students must
reinforce and role model the importance of reading on early childhood
development. Nursing education stands to benefit greatly from literacy-
promoting initiatives through greater preparation and increased skill
sets in prospective students. Higher literacy levels result in students
with greater capacity for understanding the complexities of education
today and may guarantee smoother assimilation into the professional
role.

Conclusion

The ultimate challenge facing American nurse educators is learning to
recognize the global reach of seemingly local problems. As part of the
global community of nurse educators, U.S. educators can use local action

to address the international problems of brain drain, the nursing faculty shortage, and poorly prepared students. Implementing these suggestions will be a demanding task, and portions of these strategies may seem too radical for practical use. However, failure to take bold action will only perpetuate the status quo in nursing education. The status quo is dysfunctional. In keeping with nursing's ethical mandates to promote social justice, improve the health of the populations, and advance the profession, nurse educators must face this ultimate challenge and begin working to implement change by thinking globally and acting locally.

REFERENCES

American Association of Colleges of Nursing. (AACN). (2003). *Faculty shortages in baccalaureate and graduate nursing programs: Scope of the problem and strategies for expanding the supply.* Retrieved July 3, 2003, from http://www.aacn.nche.edu/Publications/WhitePapers/FacultyShortages.htm

American Nurses Association. (2001). *Code of ethics for nurses with interpretive statements.* Retrieved September 10, 2005, from http://www.nursingworld.org/ethics/ecode/

Anders, R. L., & Kunaviktikul, W. (1999). Nursing in Thailand. *Nursing and Health Sciences, 1*, 235–239.

Baer, J. D., Cook, A. L., & Baldi, S. (2006, January). *The literacy of America's college students.* Washington, DC: American Institute for Research. Retrieved January 20, 2006, from http://www.pewtrusts.com/pubs/

Berlin, L. E., & Sechrist, K. R. (2002). The shortage of doctorally prepared nursing faculty: A dire situation. *Nursing Outlook, 50,* 50–56.

Bosch, X. (2003). Brain drain robbing Europe of its brightest young scientists. *The Lancet, 361,* 2210.

Brendtro, M., & Hegge, M. (2000). Nursing faculty: One generation away from extinction? *Journal of Professional Nursing, 16,* 97–103.

Bronstein, P. (2001). Older women in academia: Contemporary history and issues. *Journal of Women's History, 12,* 184–201.

Buchan, J. (2001). Nurses moving across borders: 'brain drain' or freedom of movement? *International Nursing Review, 48,* 65–67.

Buchan, J., & Calman, L. (2004). *The global shortage of registered nurses: An overview of issues and action.* Geneva, Switzerland: International Council of Nurses. Retrieved September 23, 2005, from http://www.icn.ch/global/shortage.pdf

Calamai, P. (2000). The three L's—Literacy and life-long learning. *An address to the Westnet 2000 Conference,* Calgary, November 2, 2000. Retrieved from http://library.nald.ca/item/364

David, B. A. (2000). Nursing's gender politics: Reformulating the footnotes. *Advances in Nursing Science, 23*(1), 83–93.

Dehghanpisheh, B. (2004, March 8). A one-way ticket. *Newsweek International* (Pacific ed.), 35.

DeYoung, S., Bliss, J., & Tracy, J. P. (2002). The nursing faculty shortage: Is there hope? *Journal of Professional Nursing, 18*, 313–319.

Emerson, R. J., & Records, K. (2005). Nursing: Profession in peril. *Journal of Professional Nursing, 21*, 9–15.

Farmer, P. (1999). The vitality of practice: On personal trajectories. In *Infections and inequalities: The modern plagues* (2nd ed., pp. 18–36). Berkeley, CA: University of California Press.

Farmer, P. (2005). *Pathologies of power: Health, human rights, and the new war on the poor.* Los Angeles: University of California Press.

Freire, P. (1970). *Pedagogy of the oppressed.* New York: Seabury.

Gladwell, M. (2002). *The tipping point: How little things can make a big difference.* Boston: Back Bay Publishers.

Glass, N. (2001). The dis-ease of nursing academia: Putting the vulnerability "out there" (Part 2). *Contemporary Nurse, 10*, 178–186.

Glass, N. (2003). Studying women nurse academics: Exposing workplace violence in Australia: Part 2. *Contemporary Nurse, 14*, 187–195.

Girot, E. A., & Enders, B. C. (2004). International educational partnership for practice: Brazil and the United States. *Journal of Advanced Nursing, 46*, 144–151.

Gordon, D. (2003). *The distribution of child poverty in the developing world: Report to UNICEF.* Bristol, UK: University of Bristol Centre for International Poverty Research.

Heinrich, K. T., Cote, J. A., Solernou, S. B., Chiffer, D. K., Bona, G. A., McKelvey, M., et al. (2003). From partners to passionate scholars: Preparing nurse educators for the new millennium. *Annual Review of Nursing Education, 1*, 109–131.

Heinrich, K. T., Pardue, K. T., Davison-Price, M., Murphy, J. I., Neese, R., Walker, P., et al. (2004). How can I help you? How can you help me? Transforming nursing education through partnerships. *Nursing Education Perspectives, 26*, 34–41.

Heinrich, K. T. (2005). Halfway between receiving and giving: A relational analysis of doctorate-prepared nurse-scholars' first 5 years after graduation. *Journal of Professional Nursing, 21*, 303–313.

Hinshaw, A. (2001, January 31). A continuing challenge: The shortage of educationally prepared nursing faculty [Electronic version]. *Online Journal of Issues in Nursing, 6*(1), manuscript 3. Retrieved February 2, 2001, from http://www.nursingworld.org/ojin/topic14/tpc14_3.htm

International Council of Nurses. (2000). *The ICN code of ethics for nurses.* Retrieved November 1, 2005, from, http://www.icn.ch/ethics.htm

International Council of Nurses. (2004, April/June). Critical situation in Paraguay. *Socio-Economic News,* No. 1, Para. 1–2. Retrieved September 23, 2005, from http://www.icn.ch/sewapr-jun04.htm

Jarrett, S. L., Hummel, F., & Whitney, K. L. (2005). Preparing for the 21st century: Graduate nursing education in Vietnam. *Nursing Education Perspectives, 26,* 172–175.

Kelly, C. M. (2002). Investing in the future of nursing education: A cry for action. *Nursing Education Perspectives, 23,* 24–29.

Ketefian, S., Daly, J., Chang, E., & Srisuphan, W. (2005). Issues and challenges in international doctoral education in nursing. *Nursing and Health Sciences, 7,* 150–156.

Kingma, M. (2001). Nursing migration: Global treasure hunt or disaster-in-the-making? *Nursing Inquiry, 8,* 205–212.

Kinsella, K., & Velkoff, V. A. (2001). *An aging world: 2001.* Retrieved October 6, 2005, fromhttp://www.nia.nih.gov/ResearchInformation/ExtramuralPrograms/Behavioral And SocialResearch/Resources.htm

Krashen, S. (2005). The "decline' of reading in America, poverty and access to books, and the use of comics in encouraging reading [Electronic version]. *Teachers' College Record.* Retrieved March 15, 2006, from http://www.tcrecord.org

Lesser, J. G., O'Neill, M. R., Burke, K. W., Scanlon, P., Hollis, K., & Miller, R. (2004). Women supporting women: A mutual aid group fosters new connections among women in midlife. *Social Work with Groups, 27,* 75–88.

Llana, S. (2006, March 6). Global stopgap for U.S. nurse deficit. *Christian Science Monitor, 3/6/06, 98,* 68.

Lopez-Claros, A., & Zahidi, S. (2006). *Women's empowerment: Measuring the global gender gap.* Geneva, Switzerland: World Economic Forum. Retrieved October 10, 2005, from http://www.weforum.org/homepublic.nsf/Content/Initiatives+subhome

Maguire, M. (2001). Beating time? The resistance, reproduction, and representation of older women in teacher education. *International Journal of Inclusive Education, 5,* 225–236.

McGivern, D. O. (2003). The scholar's nursery. *Nursing Outlook, 51,* 59–64.

Meleis, A. (2003). Brain drain or empowerment? *Journal of Nursing Scholarship, 35*(2), 105.

Mish, F. C. (Ed.). (2001). *Merriam-Webster's collegiate dictionary* (10th ed.). Springfield, MA: Merriam-Webster.

National League for Nursing. (2002). Position statement: The preparation of nurse educators. *Nursing Education Perspectives, 23,* 267–269.

National strategies wanted to plug the brain drain. (2004). *The Lancet, 364,* 556.

Neese, R. (2003). A transformational journey from clinician to educator. *Journal of Continuing Education in Nursing, 34,* 258–262.

Nunes, C. A. A., & Gaibel, E. (2002). Development of multimedia materials. In W. D. Haddad & A. Draxler (Eds.), *Technologies for education: Potentials, parameters and prospects* (pp. 134–143). Washington, DC/Paris: AED/UNESCO.

Nutbeam, D. (2000). Health literacy as a public goal: A challenge for contemporary health education and communication strategies into the 21st century. *Health Promotion International, 15*(3), 183–184.

Ortin, E. L. (1990). The brain drain as viewed by an exporting country. *International Nursing Review, 37*, 340–344.

Pang, T., Lansang, M., & Haines, A. (2002). Brain drain and health professionals. *British Medical Journal, 324*, 7336.

Peck, W., Flower, L., & Higgins, L. (1995). Community literacy. *College Composition and Communication, 46*(2), 199–222.

Reach Out and Read. (2003). *How ROR works.* Retrieved March 10, 2006, from http://www.reachoutandread.org/about how.html.

Roberts, S. J. (2000). Development of a positive professional identity: Liberating oneself from the oppressor within. *Advances in Nursing Science, 22*(4), 71–82.

Shanahan, M. (2005, September 7). *Universities 'can help offset brain drain from south.'* Retrieved September 19, 2005, from http://www.scidev.net/content/news/eng/universities-can-help-offset-brain-drain-from-south.cfm

Sigma Theta Tau International. (2003). *Arista 3—Nurses and health: A global future.* Indianapolis, IN: STTI. Retrieved August 22, 2005, from http://www.nursingsociety.org/programs/ARISTA info.htm

United Nations Educational Scientific and Cultural Organization. (2004). *World Education Report.* Paris: UNESCO.

United Nations Educational Scientific and Cultural Organization. (2005). *World Literacy Day facts.* Retrieved November 27, 2005, from http://www.uis.unesco.org

Wilbright, W. A., Haun, D. E., Romano, T., Krutzfeld, T., Fontenot, C. E., & Nolan, T. E. (2006). Computer use in an urban university hospital: Technology ahead of literacy. *CIN: Computers, Informatics, Nursing, 24*, 37–43.

Women in Literacy. (2005). *International facts.* Retrieved November 27, 2005, from http://www.womeninliteracy.org/facts.html

World Bank Group. (2001). *Intergenerational effects: The education of adults contributes to the education of children.* Retrieved September 20, 2005, from http://www1.worldbank.org/education/adultoutreach/investing.intergen.asp

Chapter 9

Using Benchmarking for Continuous Quality Improvement in Nursing Education

Diane M. Billings

F aculty in a nursing program subscribe to a testing service to identify how well their students are attaining learning outcomes for
pharmacology with the intent of revising the way the pharmacology content is presented in the curriculum; they compare their students'
results to the mean in the testing service databank. A school of nursing
wants to know how it compares with others in the state in the number of degrees conferred at 4-year colleges and universities. A research-
intensive school of nursing is preparing a report to document need for
salary increases for its faculty and reviews salary data from other schools
of nursing designated as research intensive. Promotion and tenure guidelines at a school of nursing require faculty to report the results of student
evaluation of teaching in comparison with those received by other faculty
at this school. All of these schools are using benchmarking to provide
answers to questions asked by a variety of stakeholders, including legis-
lators, institutions, peers, parents, and colleagues. These questions may
be about educational programs, teaching and learning, use of resources,
admission and graduation rates, effectiveness of online courses, and myr-
iad other indicators of successful processes and practices at their school.
This chapter describes benchmarking, a process that provides answers
to questions such as these.

This chapter was accepted on March 30, 2006.

Benchmarking

Benchmarking is the process of identifying processes or practices from other organizations or institutions and then using them to help an organization improve similar processes or practices (Alstete, 2006; American Productivity and Quality Center, 2006; Bender & Shuh, 2002; Trimble, 2006). *Benchmarks* are the measure of a best practice; *benchmarking* is the process of identifying benchmarks and applying them for performance improvement.

Benchmarking answers questions such as the following:

- How are we doing in comparison with other schools?
- What are the best practices for a given process?
- Who is using the best practices and what can we learn from them?
- What makes those schools with best practices successful?

Although results of benchmarking are useful to provide data-driven responses to stakeholders, benchmarking, as a process, is even more useful in guiding quality improvement in a variety of areas of concern to nurse educators.

Types of Benchmarking

There are at least four types of benchmarking practices used in higher education (Doerfel & Ruben, 2002; Trimble, 2006):

1. internal
2. competitive
3. generic
4. longitudinal.

Internal Benchmarking

Internal benchmarking refers to comparisons between or among departments or schools within the university. Internal benchmarking might be used to assess salary equity, compare faculty rank/tenure status among academic departments, indicate student satisfaction with teaching practices across disciplines, compare student admission/progression rates, or identify which academic unit or department is using university resources such as libraries or computing services. These findings give broad guidelines to academic units or departments as to where they stand in comparison with others in relatively similar circumstances. Internal benchmarking, therefore, provides useful data for institutional planning, as well as improving processes and outcomes in academic departments.

Competitive Benchmarking

Competitive benchmarking involves comparisons with "competitors" such as other schools of nursing. Competitive benchmarking examines processes that make competitors successful in an area of interest. Competitive benchmarking is useful when the goal is to improve a particular practice or process by learning from successful organizations.

Generic Benchmarking

Generic benchmarking examines general processes, practices, and procedures of similar schools who are not necessarily competitors. Schools of nursing use generic benchmarking to identify best practices for preparing students for licensing examinations or to determine student learning outcomes in subject areas taught in a nursing curriculum.

Longitudinal Benchmarking

Longitudinal benchmarking refers to tracking results over time. In some instances, processes, practices, or outcomes are understood in a long-term context, particularly when instituting change or when trend data will be more useful. Longitudinal benchmarking provides this view.

Benchmarking Process

Benchmarking is a process that involves a set of sequential steps. Although the process should be tailored for specific needs, the following steps are common to most benchmarking activities:

1. *Identify the area, performance, process, or practice of interest.* The area may be identified as a point of data gathering for reporting comparisons, or it may be an area identified as needing improvement.
2. *Define the benchmarks.* In this step, best practices or ideal processes are delineated, and boundaries are set around the area to be described. For example, when benchmarking faculty salaries, the salaries for tenured faculty may be the only area of interest.
3. *Determine the type of benchmarking process appropriate to elicit required data.* In this step, the educator identifies if benchmarking will involve internal comparisons, comparisons with competitors, or more general measures, such as comparisons with a general pool of data from like schools. At this point, it is important to be clear about the purpose of benchmarking and choose the appropriate approach.
4. *Identify the benchmarking peers or partners.* Here, the educator examines the characteristics of the peer or partner to match with those appropriate for the process or practice being benchmarked. For example, possible characteristics could include funding base (private vs. public school of nursing), type of program (doctoral vs. associate degree program), mission (research vs. teaching), or region (West Coast vs. southern states). At this step, it is important to choose peers carefully, matching characteristics as closely as possible; otherwise, results will be skewed and not serve the intended purpose.
5. *Gather information/performance data.* There are several ways to obtain data. One way is to subscribe to a benchmarking service that collects data in the area of interest from peer schools and provides access to a data set with a variety of characteristics that can be matched according to needs. Another way to gather data is to participate in institutional surveys conducted by the college or university. Often, these data can be reported for a specific school of nursing; some institutional research offices have a fee for this reporting; others provide the data as a service to the academic departments. Finally, it is possible for a faculty or school of nursing to develop its own surveys, questionnaires, or conduct interviews (Secor, 2002). Often, department, school, or institutional data already are being collected. For example,

student evaluation of courses and faculty teaching can be aggregated to provide a data pool from which internal benchmarking data can then be drawn.

6. *Analyze data.* At this step, data are retrieved, usually in a report that provides statistical information, such as mean, standard deviation, and range. Reports from benchmarking services often provide pictorial representation of data that make interpretation easier. The key to analyzing data is to look for gaps between the results and the benchmark. Data analysis requires careful reflection and interpretation in the specific context of the data user. Data users must understand their strengths and areas for improvement in terms of their goals and resources. Not all information will be useful, and not all practices can be adopted or adapted.

7. *Use data for improvement.* The real benefit of benchmarking lies in the ability to use benchmarking data for improvement. At this stage, dialogue is important, and key stakeholders must be involved. Senior management also should be involved as system level changes may be required to facilitate the required improvement (American Productivity and Quality Center, 2006). Identifying action steps, setting priorities, establishing deadlines, and being clear about outcomes of change occur at this time.

8. *Evaluate results.* The final step of the benchmarking process is to evaluate the outcomes. Benchmarking is a continuous process, and educators must determine the extent to which change has occurred and the effectiveness of interventions.

Integrating Benchmarking Into Education Practice

Benchmarking as a process and a tool can be integrated into education practices at schools of nursing. Benchmarking for quality improvement can be conducted at various levels of the school of nursing, including at the institutional level, the school/department level, the course level, or by individual faculty who are improving their own careers in the areas of teaching, research, or service.

At the *institutional level* (campus or university), nurse educators should be familiar with the types of institutional data that are collected.

For example, are nursing students and faculty included in the data collection? Can specific questions about nursing be added to the survey? Are results available to schools and faculty? Is there a fee to have access to these data? How can the data collected by the college, university, or health care organization be used for planning academic programs or improving programs, teaching, or student learning? Reports from institutional-level data provide guidance for areas of improvement within the school of nursing in the context of the goals of the larger university.

At the *program level*, benchmarked data can be used to improve program outcomes. For example, schools of nursing use reports from licensing and certification examinations to identify the extent to which overall program outcomes have been obtained. If pass rates are not comparable with that of peer institutions, faculty have data on which to base discussions about curriculum and/or program revision. Several commercial benchmarking services provide targeted information about common program outcomes such as "professionalism" or data from employer surveys that indicate the employment readiness for the graduates. These reports provide concrete data for areas needing change and improvement.

At the *course level,* faculty use data from nationally normed examinations in a content area or from report services from the licensing examination. Using these data, faculty can determine which courses or content areas may need improvement.

Benchmarking data can be used by *individual faculty* members to improve their own teaching, research, or service components of their faculty role. Although most faculty are accustomed to receiving student ratings of their course and teaching, many schools of nursing use university testing services to aggregate student evaluations of all courses and instruction and can report means, standard deviations, and percentages for grouped data at the school or university level. Faculty can then understand how students perceive their own course and instruction in terms of the school or college benchmarks.

Faculty who are teaching online courses for the first time, for example, find it helpful to have benchmarks for best practices to guide implementation and revision of their courses (Billings, Connors, & Skiba, 2001). Research-intensive faculty can use numbers and dollar amounts of grants and numbers of their publications, compared with others in similar circumstances, as benchmarks for guiding the development of a career as a researcher.

The Culture of Evidence

Using benchmarking approaches in schools of nursing is facilitated in a "culture of evidence" (Hedges, 2006). This culture exists when there is an expectation that the work of students, faculty, and administrators is reviewed and continuously improves. The culture is fostered by respect for each faculty's contribution to the mission of the school, clarity about goals, and open dialogue that fosters reflection and direction.

Developing and maintaining a culture of evidence is the responsibility of all stakeholders. Students become a part of the culture when faculty orients them at the beginning of the program about their role in providing helpful feedback to all aspects of the academic program, and continue to reinforce this message throughout the program. Faculty contribute to the culture through honest and open communication, articulating the goals and benchmarks that are to be attained, and providing helpful peer review in the context of improvement. Also, faculty have responsibilities to respond to findings from benchmarking reports and communicate intended changes and improvements to the stakeholders. Administrators support the culture by removing "blame," using data rather than opinion to guide change; celebrating improvement; and maintaining an environment in which improvement is the norm.

Summary

Benchmarking is a method and a tool for assessing practices and processes for the purpose of continuous quality improvement. The process is systematic, and nurse educators must understand the benchmarks, how data are collected, who are the peer partners, and the data that are analyzed. Also, faculty need to be involved in the dialogue at all points of the process. With this information at hand, educators can make decisions about changing practices within their own setting. Benchmarking in and of itself can prompt a "culture of evidence" with the end goal of improvement of the practices, processes, and outcomes for a variety of stakeholders. Without dialogue among all stakeholders, opportunities for improvement are lost in the benchmarking reports.

REFERENCES

Alstete, J. (2006). Benchmarking in higher education: Adapting best practices to improve quality. Retrieved March 1, 2006, from http://www.ericdigests.org/1997-3/bench.html

American Productivity and Quality Center. (2006). Knowledge Sharing Network. Retrieved March 1, 2006, from http://www.apqc.org/portal/apqc/ksn?paf_gear_id

Bender, B., & Schuh, J. (2002). Editor's notes. In B. Bender & J. Schuh (Eds.), *Using benchmarking to inform practice in higher education*. San Francisco: Jossey-Bass.

Billings, D., Connors, H., & Skiba, D. (2001). Benchmarking best practices in web-based nursing courses. *Advances in Nursing Science, 23*(3), 41–52.

Doerfel, M., & Ruben, B. (2002). J. (Eds). *Using benchmarking to inform practice in higher education*. San Francisco: Jossey-Bass.

Hedges, L. V. (2006). *The culture of evidence*. Retrieved March 27, 2006, from http://www.meetinglink.org/mspnetwork/Mtg2Papers/MSPPI_MeetingCultureofEvidence.doc

Secor, R. (2002). Penn State joins the Big Ten and learns to benchmark. In B. Bender & J. Schuh (Eds). *Using benchmarking to inform practice in education* (pp. 65–78). San Francisco: Jossey-Bass.

Trimble, D. (2006). *Benchmarking—Uncovering best practices and learning from others*. Retrieved March 1, 2006, from http://www.procsi.com/benchmarking.htm

Part III

Enhancing Learning and Student Development Through Technology and Assessment

Chapter 10

Student Support Services for Distance Education Students in Nursing Programs

Ramona Nelson

D istance education has become an increasingly effective tool in meeting the educational needs of students seeking degrees in nursing. A quality online education program requires a well-designed and well-delivered curriculum, as well as a wide range of student support services. Examples of key student support services include academic advising, bookstore services, financial aid, and library services. This chapter describes required online student support services. It explains how online student support services can be structured and identifies a number of resources for developing these services.

Growth of Distance Education in Nursing

Over the last decade, higher education has seen a rapid growth of distance education. In the 2000–2001 academic year, 56% (2,320) of all 2-year and 4-year Title IV-eligible, degree-granting institutions, offered distance education courses for any level or audience. In addition, 12% of all institutions indicated that they planned to start offering distance education courses in the next 3 years (U.S. Department of Education, National Center for Educational Statistics, 2003). On many campuses, nurses have been the leaders in establishing distance education

---

This chapter was accepted on April 6, 2006.

programs. Johnson & Johnson Health Care Systems, Inc., maintains a comprehensive online searchable database of nursing programs in the United States at http://www.discovernursing.com. In March 2006, a search of this database for online programs produced 80 hits. Each hit was a college or university offering one or more distance education nursing programs.

Along with the growth of distance education, there has been a growth in the literature related to this topic. A search of the Cumulative Index of Nursing and Allied Health Literature (CINAHL) from 1996 to 2000, using the keyword "distance education," produced 160 hits. The same search for the next 5-year interval produced 265 hits. Clearly, much is happening in distance education and more specifically much is happening in nursing educational programs. However, a search of both CINAHL and MEDLINE (1966–March 2006) combining the keywords ("distance education" *and* "student support services") resulted in a total of only three hits (Fraser, 1998; Allen & Nero, 1999; Walker, 1990). All three of these publications written in the 1990s noted that student support services were important to distance education, but provided little additional information about these types of services.

Why Provide Online Student Support Services?

Why should student support services be provided for distance education students? The answer to this question may seem obvious. Failure to provide quality student support services can decrease learning achievement, learner satisfaction, and most likely increase attrition (Harrington, Laster, Stennet, & Carnwell, 2001). On the other hand, high-quality online student services can help in recruiting students, facilitate degree completion, as well as establish and maintain an active alumni (Brigham, 2001). Most universities, "recognizing the important role that student services play in learner success and retention, have a full range of student services in place to support their on-campus learners. Yet, many have failed to provide the same level of service to their off-campus learners who cannot come to campus" (Shea & Armitage, n.d., p. 2).

The reason for this failure most likely relates to how and where distance education programs have developed. Many of these programs have developed within specific disciplines or continuing education units. The focus was on developing the courses and programs, as well as preparing the faculty. Support services were often added only when the need for a specific service became obvious. For example, the bookstore might be asked to ship textbooks to off-campus students. Often, these types of requests required that the departments providing these support services make changes in well-established policies and procedures that were effectively meeting the needs of on-campus students. On many campuses, this has resulted in duplicate systems, supporting a limited number of distance education students, compared with the traditional students. Not only are the various departments providing student support now being asked to provide services for distance education students, but they are also being asked to provide those services online.

Guidelines from professional organizations, as well as individual authors, stress the importance of providing online student services to distance education students. However, for traditional universities, one of the most important motivations for developing online student services is the value of online student services to the traditional student. Table 10.1 lists a number of university academic services that are provided online for both traditional and distance education students. The traditional student's first impression of a campus is often created by that institution's Web page. If that first experience is convenient, efficient, and student centered, students will have a positive impression. However, if the student must search across several departments and in the end find a virtual run around of inconsistent and outdated information, their first impression is negative (Shea, 2005). For the distance education student who never expects to come on campus, this may be their only impression. Because student services are often provided by a variety

TABLE 10.1   University Academic Services for Traditional and Distance Education Students

Service	Types of Services
Admissions	Requests for information and online applications
Registration	Course catalog, course schedule, and available "seats"
Financial aid	Online application forms and scholarship information
Student accounts	Statement of charges and option to pay online
Student records	Access to transcripts, grades, and degree audits
Student ID	Ability to edit demographic data

of departments across the university, they—more than any other area of the university—are most at risk of creating such an impression.

However, putting all student services online will not eliminate the need for support services specifically designed for distance education students. This was demonstrated by Harrington and colleagues (2001), who compared the academic learning support needs of two groups of nursing and allied health students. One group was campus based, and the other group was distance learning based. Although there was significant overlap in the types of services needed, there were also differences. In addition, the distance education students had higher expectations for the support provided. Shea and Armitage (n.d.) listed a number of these types of expectations. These expectations with examples are described in Table 10.2. The emphasis in this chapter is on the support services of significant concern for online nursing students.

Although there is recognition of the importance of student support services for online nursing students, the question can be raised: Why should nursing faculty be concerned with these services? After all, are not nursing faculty already busy with developing online courses and advising these online learners? Because the nursing faculty deal directly with these online students as teachers and advisors, in the final analysis

TABLE 10.2   Examples of Student Expectations for Online Student Services

Expectation	Explanation
Self service	Let me do it online 24/7 and not have to call or contact someone.
Just-in-time	Tell me what I need to know when I need to know. For example, provide me a link to the library orientation when I have a library assignment.
Push selections	Send me reminders such as registration deadlines when I need them.
Personalized	Do not send me information about food service options if I do not live on campus.
Integrated	If I register for too few credits, send me an alert that this will impact my financial aid.
Student-centered Web-designed pages	Include a link to the bookstore when I register for courses, even if these are different departments in the university.

they are the best advocates for ensuring students receive the university services needed for their success.

Whereas this chapter provides an introduction to needed online support services, each nursing program and each university must customize these services to their setting and their population. For example, in some cases, distance education students can also be on campus. WSU Online, the online campus of Weber State University located in Utah, determined that 78% of their distance education students were also taking courses on campus (Smith, 2001). Their approach to providing online student services reflects this reality as demonstrated at http://wsuonline.weber.edu/students/studentresources/services.htm. In contrast, all students at Excelsior College are off campus. Their approach to support services reflects this reality as demonstrated at https://www.excelsior.edu/.

Types of Student Support Services

Assessment and Evaluation for Online Learning

From the student perspective, support services start with an opportunity to determine if they can expect to have a successful learning experience with distance education. Several online sites provide both survey and reflective questions that students can use to make this decision. Distance Education Clearinghouse, which is managed and produced by the University of Wisconsin—Extension, provides a portal to several such sites. This is located at http://www.uwex.edu/disted/students.html. These sites can help the student determine if:

- their learning style and study habits are congruent with distance education learning
- they have the needed technical skills to succeed in a distance education program
- they have the reading comprehension and related literacy skills to succeed
- they have the financial resources to support their education
- their level of motivation provides the potential to complete a distance education course/program, and
- the program or institution is accredited or otherwise recognized.

Several of the sites that provide these assessment tools and resources also provide related support services, as well as other resources to find appropriate learning opportunities. These types of services are most effective if they are integrated with the recruitment and orientation materials that have been developed for a specific program. An excellent example of this approach is provided by The School of Nursing at Georgia Southwestern State University. The URL for this example is http://www.gsw.edu/~son/Distance.html.

Orientation

Like all students, distance education students must be oriented to the university, their educational program, and their courses. Because different areas of the university are involved with each of these three areas, the student orientation for distance education students can easily become disorganized with key components missing. To avoid these problems, the orientation should be carefully organized from the prospective of the students' experience and learning.

University Orientation. Orientation to the university can be divided into two areas. First is the university as an institution. It is this orientation that creates credibility for the university as a quality educational institution and is the beginning of creating a committed alumnus. These orientation materials can often be developed with general recruitment materials that help to control the cost and keep materials current. The orientation should include the type of institution (e.g., community college or major research institution) it is, a brief history, its mission, its size, accreditation information, and an introduction to key administrators. A virtual tour can be effective in creating a sense of presence for the university.

The second area of university orientation is an orientation to the various support services offered to distance education students. As demonstrated in this chapter, universities provide a wide range of services for distance education students. But how are students to know what services are available and how to access these when needed? The "dumping down" approach of providing information on any and all services is not effective. When this approach is used, few students actually look at these materials and those that do soon forget the details.

Organization of the Web pages can help to lead students to the services at the point of need. In addition, some services require more extensive orientation. The best example is the online library services for distance education students. The more extensive orientations are more likely to be accessed and used if they are integrated into the course orientation.

Program Orientation. This level of orientation introduces the distance education student to their school or department, as well as the specific education program they have selected. It is helpful if this orientation follows the same format as the university orientation with information about the mission, history, and types of nursing programs offered. In addition, the orientation should include Web pages with information about the individual nursing administrators and faculty. It is helpful if these Web sites are not limited to a sterile bio, but also include pictures and some general personal information.

Technology Support

Technology support for distance education should be designed for prospective students considering a distance education program, as well as current students taking distance education courses within the university. The actual screen design and navigation should be integrated with the overall recruitment and online orientation programs designed for the distance education students. Three questions guide the technology related content to be included within these pages:

1. What hardware, software, and Internet connectively do I need?
2. How can I be sure I have the technology to succeed?
3. How do I get help when the technology does not function as planned or I do not know what to do?

Hardware, Software, and Internet Connectivity. Depending on what is required, four types of hardware requirements may be needed. First, students will need to know if the program can be completed with either a PC or Mac-based computer. If both types of computers can be used, students will next need to know both the minimum and recommended requirements for both types of computers. The minimum requirements are used to decide if the student's current computer is satisfactory. The recommended requirements are used as a guide if the student needs to purchase a new computer. Software requirements should also include minimum and recommended versions of all software, including spyware, virus checker, and plug-ins. It is helpful if the screen with this information is linked to site(s) for downloading needed plug-ins and software that will be provided by the university as well as a site offering academic prices for required software. Although these details should be provided, it is important to appreciate that many potential students will need additional help determining if they have the needed technology.

In the end, the question, "How can I be sure I have the technology I need?," is best answered with a "browser test." A browser test lets potential students actually test their computer and provides feedback on what is needed. An excellent example of this approach, as well as how the technical requirements can be configured in a user-friendly way, is demonstrated by Duquesne University at http://www.distancelearning. duq.edu/prospective/overview.cfm?DivID=01.

Finally, the technical requirements should explain the level of Internet connectivity required, as well as the related Internet support services provided by the university. For example, does the university provide a toll-free number for a dial-in modem pool or are all students required to arrange their Internet connectivity via an Internet service provider? Currently, most distance education programs can still be accessed via a dial-in connection. However, broadband connectively, such as cable or DSL, is becoming important. If this level of connectivity is required, students should have this information before applying to the university.

Ongoing Support. Although distance education technology and software have become much more reliable, distance education students continue to need ongoing technical support. The scope of support provided can be outlined with four questions. These are:

1. *What level of support will be provided for equipment and services that are not provided or not under the control of the university?* For example, if a student is planning to access the course management software from his place of employment and is experiencing a technical problem because of a firewall, should the university's technical support contact the technical support at the place of employment?

2. *How should support services be organized from the student's prospective?* The university is attempting to support: (1) hardware; (2) a variety of software; (3) e-mail, connectivity, and network issues; (4) course management software; and (5) in many cases, passwords for these different services. Students would like to have one portal for all support, but it can be difficult for technical staff to be prepared to troubleshoot such a broad range of support services. This can mean that students may need to access different support services for different technical problems. In many cases, faculty become the gatekeeper helping students navigate access to needed support services.

3. *What are the hours of support?* Distance education students often work on their classes during off hours and weekends. Technical problems can be especially frustrating if the student has set aside a block of time and now cannot get into their course and cannot obtain help with their problem. Students prefer that technical support be there 24/7 and ready when they need it. However, the demand for support is not evenly distributed across the 24/7 time period or the term. Demand is much higher when (1) there have been upgrades or changes in the university technology; (2) the beginning of the term when students are still setting up and learning the software; and (3) during high usage periods, such as midterm and finals. However, providing 24/7 support for all areas of potential support throughout the term can be very expensive.

4. *What is the format of the support?* There are five options that can be used to provide most of the support that any student might need. These approaches are not either/or options, but can be mixed and matched to the hours of support. The first approach is to provide a Web site with answers to frequently asked questions or approaches to common problems. The second option is to provide automated support for selected services such as resetting passwords. The third approach is to provide e-mail support, with the e-mails triaged to the staff most prepared to handle the problem. A fourth option is to provide technical support via instant messaging or chat. Finally, the fifth approach is toll-free phone support can be used to deal with technical problems. The more personal the service, the higher the cost to the university.

Advising

Academic Advising. Online nursing students are often goal-directed with plans for additional education beyond the current program. Completion of the current program and preparation for additional study frequently frame the goals of the advising process. Academic advising in the online environment requires a systematic process of providing the student with academic direction while building a relationship with that student. The advisor is a coach that keeps the student moving forward to achieve his/her goals.

The online advising process benefits from structure. Ideally, the advisor is assigned when the student is admitted and hopefully follows that student throughout the total program. Academic advising materials should include a clear description of all program requirements, course requirements, and requirements for graduation. The advisors' role is to help the student plan a program of studies that matches: (1) the course and graduation requirements, (2) the advisee's long-term career goals, (3) the course and credit options, and (4) the students' availability to take courses. Figure 10.1 demonstrates an example of a survey sent to advisees before developing their program of studies. Figure 10.2 is an example of an online form for developing a program of studies.

Although online nursing students have many responsibilities that often require revisions in a program of studies, this should be a written document that the advisee and advisor can follow and revise as needed. Once the program of studies has been established, the advisor should contact his/her advisee on a regular basis, with this contact occurring at least once a term before registration for the next term. In many cases, building an effective advising relationship requires more frequent contact. This is especially true during the first semester and just before the last semester of the students nursing program.

Tutoring. Online students may need tutorial help with specific courses, specific skills (e.g., writing), or they may need general study skills specific to distance education learning. Online peer tutors can be especially helpful in selected courses. For example, students often appreciate a tutor when taking statistics. If tutors are not available, a "study buddy" can be helpful. It may seem obvious that the study buddy should be a student who is doing well in the course. However, students in a distance education course may not always know which classmate would be

RN- BSN Advisee Survey

Name:

How many classes do you want to take per semester?

Do you want to take summer classes?

I am interested in the following electives

☐ **NURS 412/413 – Nursing Process with School Populations**
(3 theory; 3 clinical). Prerequisite: NURS 313/314 Placement - Junior/Senior Level
☐ **NURS 415 – Management of School Health Services**
Prerequisite: Enrollment in school nursing or permission of instructor
☐ **NURS 429 – Financial Management for Nursing Case Managers**
(3 semester hours)
☐ **NURS 450 – Health Care Informatics Internship**
(3 credits)
☐ **NURS 498A – Trends in Nursing Care of Children**
☐ **NURS 498 – Nursing Care of the Older Adult**
☐ **NURS 498 C – Nursing and Contemporary Women's Health Issues**
☐ **NURS 510 – Cardiovascular Function: Assessment and Treatment**
Prerequisites: Human Anatomy and Physiology or permission of the instructor.
☐ **NURS 511 – Advanced Healthcare Informatics**
Prerequisite: NURS 311 or permission of instructor

☐ I am interested in a minor or special certificate:
Options:
☐ Healthcare informatics minor   ☐ Case Management Certificate
☐ School Nurse Certificate   ☐ Gerontology Certificate

My admission letter said I needed liberal studies credits: ☐ Yes   ☐ No
If Yes, Please tell me some interests that you have so that we can look for courses that you would enjoy.

My plans after graduation include:

FIGURE 10.1   Sample advisee survey.
Source: Initial form designed by Kerry Risco (kerry.risko@sru.edu) and revised by Ramona Nelson (ramona.nelson@sru.edu). Reprinted by permission, April 12, 2006.

a good potential study buddy. Faculty intervention can be key in helping the student establish a study buddy relationship.

An online writing center is another type of tutoring service that is valued by distance education students. Nurses are often nontraditional students returning to school after a period of time when they were not

SLIPPERY ROCK UNIVERSITY OF PENNSYLVANIA
RN-BSN PROGRAM
INDIVIDUAL PROGRAM PLAN

Name of Student: ____

Date ____

Expected Date of Graduation: ____

Advisor Name: ____

Minors:
____
____
____

Certificates:
____
____
____

Year 1 Course #	Credits	Fall Term, 20____ Name	Year 1 Course #	Credits	Spring Term, 20____ Name	Year 1 Course #	Summer Term, 20____ Name	Credits
	____			____				____
	____			____				____
	____			____				____
	____			____				____

Year 2 Course #	Credits	Fall Term, 20____ Name	Year 2 Course #	Credits	Spring Term, 20____ Name	Year 2 Course #	Summer Term, 20____ Name	Credits
	____			____				____
	____			____				____
	____			____				____
	____			____				____

Year 3 Course #	Credits	Fall Term, 20____ Name	Year 3 Course #	Credits	Spring Term, 20____ Name	Year 3 Course #	Summer Term, 20____ Name	Credits
	____			____				____
	____			____				____
	____			____				____
	____			____				____

Year 4 Course #	Credits	Fall Term, 20____ Name	Year 4 Course #	Credits	Spring Term, 20____ Name	Year 4 Course #	Summer Term, 20____ Name	Credits
	____			____				____
	____			____				____
	____			____				____
	____			____				____

NURS 415 – Spring term
NURS 412/413 – Fall term
NURS 511 – Fall term

NURS 510 – Fall term
NURS 429 – Spring term
NURS 498 – Spring term

Statistical Methods – Summer and Fall terms
Medical Ethics – Summer term
Special Education – Summer term

FIGURE 10.2 Sample program of studies.

Source: Designed by the nursing faculty at Slippery Rock University. Reprinted by permission, April 12, 2006.

required to use formal writing skills. In addition, for several years, they may have been using the concise abbreviated writing style of nursing documentation. These students can benefit from help with form and style as well as help with concise clear sentence structure. However, these types of services take time. The student must first produce a document, and the tutor must then have time to review and provide feedback on that document. The process may take several iterations. Therefore, requiring first drafts and establishing early due dates within specific courses are very helpful in ensuring that students are able to access these types of online services.

Novice online learners also need help with study skills for online learning. One approach is to establish a Web page with links to various resources and tools. The site can be used as part of the orientation or as a referral resource for students who need some assistance with online study skills. An excellent example of a Web site demonstrating study skills for distance education can be found at http://www.westga .edu/~online/.

Online learning skills can also be integrated into the first online course(s) in the curriculum. For example, online learners frequently need help with basic computer skills, such as setting up folders, organizing bookmarks in a browser, or installing required plug-ins. In addition, they are learning how to navigate through the technology and course management software used to deliver distance education. At the same time they are learning to organize and study content that has not been delivered via a traditional lecture. Many of these students have made personal and financial adjustments to return to school and as a result, they may have a fair amount of anxiety about their decision.

As students make these adjustments and become comfortable with distance education learning the following techniques are helpful:

- Structure the first couple of classes in the course around basic skills, such as use of plug-ins or organizing bookmarks
- Include an orientation to the technical support services as part of the first classes in the first course
- Encourage students to answer each other's questions on a discussion board
- Have students use an online discussion board to share their anxieties

- Reassure students that faculty members understand and accept these concerns
- Provide sample assessment experiences, such as sample online quizzes, before students use online assessments for actual grades.

Creating Online Peer Networks

In traditional classroom settings, students quickly become acquainted and develop important friendships. These social networks and friendships are an important part of the students' support systems during their student days and long after they have graduated. However, the development of these social networks does not occur as spontaneously in a distance education environment. Learning experiences with specific courses can be designed to encourage the development of social networks. However additional support can be required to maintain these networks after the course is completed.

To meet this need, a course management software shell can be used to establish an online student union. At Slippery Rock University, the online student union is called the BSN Forum. New nursing students are enrolled in the BSN Forum as soon as they are admitted to the program. The BSN Forum includes links to all other student services, orientation materials, the student handbook and each of the forms that a student might need for school-related activities. The students are encouraged to become familiar with the materials in the BSN Forum while they are learning how to navigate around the course management software. This is the beginning of their orientation to the program.

In addition, several discussion forums have been established. Some examples include a forum for selling books, a forum for humor, and a discussion about which courses should be taken or not taken at the same time. There is also a forum for posting jobs and educational opportunities as well as a forum on "important developments in health care." Key reports or announcements are posted in this forum and students are encouraged to comment.

One of the early learning activities in their first online course is to post a homepage in the BSN Forum. Again, they are encouraged to look around and to become acquainted with other students in the program. They often discover other students they have met before enrolling at Slippery Rock University. Because all students are enrolled, an e-mail can be sent to any and all groups of students.

E-mail sent via the BSN Forum is highly effective when the faculty or a student needs to get a message to all students in the program. For example, the student representative to the nursing faculty committee sends an e-mail a week before each meeting asking for student comments or concerns. When the nursing program was last visited by the National League for Nursing Accreditation Commission, e-mail and the discussion forum in the BSN Forum were used to provide the visitors with access to the students.

It should be noted that an online student union requires maintenance. Old postings must be removed. New reports and ideas need to be generated. New procedures, policies, and links need to be added as they develop. Each year, a specific faculty person assumes this responsibility. This can be conceptualized as being the advisor to the student government.

Library

The Board of Directors of the Association of College and Research Libraries approved *Guidelines for Distance Learning Library Services* in June 2004. These guidelines are available at http://www.ala.org/ala/acrl/acrlstandards/guidelinesdistancelearning.htm and provide an excellent resource for planning and assessing online library resources. Library resources needed to support online nursing programs include the collection or content used to support the nursing program, reference library support services, and the instructional services.

Library Collection. The collection within a library can exist in any media from hardcopy books to film. In this discussion related to support for online learning, the emphasis is on online access to nursing books and journals. The specific nursing-related collection selected by an individual library depends on the nursing programs being offered by the college or university. For example, if a university offered an online graduate program with a focus in nursing administration, one would expect to find a more comprehensive collection related to administration and research than might be expected if the university offered an RN completion program only. In all cases, the faculty members need to work closely with the librarian in selecting materials for the collection. A key resource for assessing any nursing library collection and planning future goals is the *Essential Nursing References*. This document, which is maintained by the Interagency Council on Information Resources for Nursing (ICIRN) can be accessed at http://www.nln.org/nlnjournal/nursingreferences1.htm. Additional information about ICIRN can be found at http://www.icirn.org/about/. Although the specific collection needed depends on the specific nursing programs offered, all online nursing programs present specific challenges.

Because the majority of nursing faculty received their education with the support of a traditional library, the first challenge is to ensure that faculty members understand the organization and process for accessing online library resources. This knowledge is necessary for the nursing faculty to participant effectively in the selection of online library resources. Online resources may be, for example, books, chapters, conference proceedings, or journals. A selected collection of these resources is aggregated into databases by vendors or organizations, such as the National Library of Medicine. MEDLINE or CINAHL are examples of literature databases in health care. These literature databases can be bibliographical, full text, or a combination. For online learners, online access to full-text materials is imperative.

Access to these databases is provided by vendors. The university library will pay a licensing fee to the vendor for access to each database. In other words, the library does not own the resource, but has purchased access for a specific time period. Licensing fees are a major expense, and the details of these contracts vary. For example, the vendor may include 50 full-text books in a collection, but the library may have only selected three. The library may have also minimized their costs by limiting the number of students who can access an online resource at the same time. Understanding how the library tracks use of online resources and the related costs is necessary to participant effectively with the library in making these types of decisions. For example, if access to a book costs $250 per year and that book is accessed five times in one year the library may decide that $50 per view or use is too expensive and eliminate that reference. In turn, faculty may shy away from using online library resources that can easily be eliminated.

As a general rule in health care, full-text literature databases consist of either books or journals and other materials. In other words, a collection of full-text books will not contain journals. Table 10.3 lists major vendors offering access to full-text journals, proceedings, and related materials. Most of these vendors offer a comprehensive database of full-text journals.

TABLE 10.3   Vendors Providing Full-Text Journal, Internet-Based Access to Nursing Journals

Vendor	URL
EBSCO Publishing	http://www.epnet.com/
ProQuest	http://www.il.proquest.com
OVID Technologies	http://www.ovid.com/

Table 10.4 lists selected vendors providing online full-text access to nursing books. The online full-text book nursing collections offered by these vendors are inadequate to support any nursing program. As a result, libraries must offer other approaches for students to access nursing books. In most cases this involves setting up a procedure where books and related materials can be sent and returned via postal mail, or materials can be copied and distributed by mail, fax, or electronically. Copyright law plays a major role in determining what can be copied and distributed. Another important consideration in developing these services is how the costs will be covered. Students may be charged directly or this might be part of the library budget.

Reference Support. Distance education students, like all students, require the support of reference librarians. There are several options that can be used to offer this service in the online environment. Well-designed "quick guides" that respond to common questions can be very helpful. However, library services are constantly changing, and these must be reviewed on a regular basis. In addition, online support can include toll-free phone numbers, chat, e-mail, and instant messaging. Key to online support is a librarian who is knowledgeable about nursing resources and understands the full use of the technology. In addition, there must be clear policies stating when reference support services are available and how long students can expect to wait for responses.

Instruction. Library-related instruction provided by university librarians can be classified into two areas. These are orientation to accessing library resources and information literacy. Online tutorials can be effective in meeting both of these needs. However, tutorials must be constantly updated and revised as library resources and services evolve.

TABLE 10.4   Vendors Providing Full-Text, Internet-Based Access to Nursing Books

Vendor	Total Nursing Books as of 7/11/06	URL and Comments
STAT!REF	22	http://www.statref.com/PDFs/Resourceby Discipline.pdf Most of the books in this database are on either the Brandon/Hill or Dooly list of recommended books.
OVID Technologies	41	http://www.ovid.com/ This vendor lists 41 books under nursing but not all of these books would be classified as nursing text by most nursing faculty.
Online Computer Library Center: Netlibrary	351	http://www.netlibrary.com/ Only 85 of these books were published in 2000 or later.
Ebrary	N/A	http://www.ebrary.com/corp/index.htm Selected nursing books published by Springer/Kluwer and Jones & Bartlett are included in the Health, Biomedical, and Clinical Sciences databases, as well as the Academic databases.

Information literacy is a special challenge for online students. Many distance education faculty, in an attempt to make distance education more convenient, provide students with all reading materials related to each course. This is a disservice to these students, because they have no opportunity to develop information literacy skills within their discipline. The American Library Association has developed information literacy standards for higher education (American Library Association, 2000). The American Nurses Association has identified information literacy as a required skill of beginning nurses (American Nurses Association Workgroup, 2001). Instruction in information literacy is best provided as a joint effort of the nursing and library faculty and integrated

TABLE 10.5   Online Resources for Teaching Information Literacy in Nursing

Resource	URL
Information Literacy Competency Standards for Higher Education	http://www.ala.org/ala/acrl/acrlstandards/ informationliteracycompetency.htm
National Forum on Information Literacy	http://www.infolit.org/members/index.html
Objectives for Information Literacy Instruction: A Model Statement for Academic Librarians	http://www.ala.org/ala/acrl/acrlstandards/ objectivesinformation.htm
Information Literacy at IUP	http://www.lib.iup.edu/infolit/infolit.html
Texas Information Literacy Tutorial	http://tilt.lib.utsystem.edu/

IUP, Indiana University of Pennsylvania.

throughout the online curriculum. Table 10.5 provides resources to support online nursing faculty in developing online information literacy learning experiences.

Additional Services

Alumni Services. Alumni can be a major resource for an online program. They can provide access to clinical settings, act as mentors for current students, be a source of prospective graduate students, and support scholarship opportunities. However, an active online program is needed to involve alumni in the institution. An example of such a program, developed by Excelsior College, can be seen by clicking on the link titled Alumni Connection, which is prominently displayed on the homepage for the college (http://www.excelsior.edu).

Bookstore. Distance education students must be able to order their books online from a secure site. The online bookstore should be able to provide this service 24/7 and ensure a timely response to requests. Not all campuses are prepared to maintain an online bookstore, and some campuses have found that outsourcing is a more effective approach (Brigham, 2001). If distance education students do not receive quality cost-effective service from the campus bookstore, they soon find other online resources for meeting their textbook needs. However, this can present problems if students purchase the wrong edition or a copy of the text that is missing passwords, CD-ROMs, or other materials. Usually, this error is not discovered until the second or even third week of class.

Distance education students cannot be required to purchase their books from the campus bookstore; even with good service, some students will elect to go elsewhere. In addition, distance education students will frequently purchase used books from other students in the program. One of the most effective ways to decrease the number of textbook problems is to post a list of all required books with related details at the time of registration for the next term.

Disability Services. Most nurses begin their nursing careers in clinical settings. These settings are not forgiving for those who develop disabilities. One of the reasons for returning to school can be the development of disabilities and the need to work in another area of nursing. In 1998, Congress amended the Rehabilitation Act to require federal agencies to make their electronic and information technology accessible to people with disabilities. Section 508 of that act was written to eliminate information technology barriers. To meet the requirements of this law, and more importantly, to meet the needs of all nursing students in distance education programs, online nursing programs must include student support services that are accessible to students with disabilities. Table 10.6 includes several links with resources for understanding the law and for designing effective Web sites and related policies.

Mediation and Conflict Resolution. Nursing programs have policies and procedures for dealing with grade appeals, discrimination concerns, and other conflicts. However, the procedures are usually designed for a traditional setting. Distance education students need to know who they can contact if they have these types of problems, and there needs to be a clear procedure for achieving fair and reasonable resolutions. An example of this type of service can be seen at http://www.athabascau.ca/studserv/ombuds.html.

TABLE 10.6   Resources for Ensuring Students With Disabilities Have Full Access

Resource	URL
Access Board is an independent Federal agency devoted to accessibility for people with disabilities	http://www.access-board.gov/
Section 508 enacted to eliminate barriers in information technology	http://www.section508.gov/
National Center on Accessible Distance Learning (AccessDL)	http://www.washington.edu/doit/
W3C: WAI: Strategies, guidelines, resources to make the Web accessible to people with disabilities	http://www.w3.org/WAI/

WAI, Web Accessibility Initiative.

TABLE 10.7   General Resources for Developing Online Student Support Services

Resource	URL
Center for Transforming Student Services	http://www.centss.org/
Principles of Good Practice for Electronically Offered Academic Degree and Certificate Programs	http://www.wcet.info/projects/balancing/principles.asp
Guidelines for Creating Student Services Online	http://www.wcet.info/projects/laap/guidelines/
Admission Policies: The Key to Success	http://www.detc.org/downloads/Occasional%20Paper11%20-%20Admissions%20Policies.pdf
DETC Student Services Handbook	http://www.detc.org/forSale.html
Online Journal of Distance Learning Administration	http://www.westga.edu/~distance/jmain11.html
Guide to Developing Online Student Services	http://www.wcet.info/resources/publications/guide/guide.htm

DETC, Distance Education and Training Council.

Conclusion

Online courses increased by 22.9% in 2003 and again by 18.2% in 2004. This growth rate is 10 times the projected rate for the higher education student body (Allen & Seaman, 2005). Given these statistics, online student services supporting distance education learning can be expected to expand in terms of the scope and depth of resources offered. As these programs grow, so will the need for high-quality student support services for distance education students. Table 10.7 offers general resources for developing these services.

Daré, Zapata, and Thomas (2005), in their research on assessing the needs of distance education students, found that more than 30% of distance learners would likely use counseling services, fitness or wellness facilities, online leadership development series, and students' health services, if they were available. As technology continues to support connectivity, nursing education should continue to advocate for more and better services for all of our students.

REFERENCES

Allen, I. E., & Seaman, J. (2005). *Growing by degrees: Online education in the United States.* Published by the Sloan Consortium. Retrieved March 19, 2006, from http://www.sloan-c.org/resources/growing_by_degrees.pdf

Allen, P., & Nero, L. (1999). Community partnerships in nursing education. *Association of Black Nursing Faculty Journal, 10*(2), 54–55.

American Library Association. (2000). *Information literacy competency standards for higher education.* Retrieved March 19, 2006, from http://www.ala.org/ala/acrl/acrlstandards/standards.pdf

American Nurses Association Workgroup (Staggers, N., Gassert, C., Kwai, J. L., Hunter, K. M., Nelson, R., Sensmeier, J., Struck, D., & Welton, J.). (2001). *Scope and standards of nursing informatics practice.* Washington, DC: American Nurses Publishing.

Brigham, D. (2001, January). Converting student support services to online delivery. *Institutional Review of Research in Open and Distance Learning* (Vol. 1, No. 2). Retrieved March 20, 2006, from http://www.irrodl.org/index.php/irrodl/article/view/23/59

Dare, L. A., Zapata, L. P., & Thomas, A. G. (2005). Assessing the needs of distance learners: A student affairs perspective. *New Directions in Students Services, 112,* 39–54.

Fraser, J. H. (1998). *Administrative issues in nursing distance education programs.* [Doctoral Dissertation Research]. University of Alberta: Canada, p. 283.

Harrington, C., Laster, D., Stennet, A., & Carnwell, R. (2001). *Diagnosing student support needs for distance education.* Retrieved March 18, 2006, from http://www.indstate. edu/oirt/inair/news/2001%20INAIR%20Presentations/CharleyHarrington_diagno se_student_disted.pdf

Shea, P. A. (2005). Serving students online: Enhancing their experience. *New Directions for Student Services, 112,* 15–24.

Shea, P. A., & Armitage, S. (n.d.). Guidelines for creating student services online. In *WCET LAAP Project beyond the administrative core: Creating web-based student services for online learners.* Retrieved March 18, 2006, from http://www.wcet.info/ projects/laap/guidelines/overview.asp

Smith, S. (2001). Beyond face-to-face: One institution's journey to develop on-line student services and ways to get started. *Students Affairs On-Line, 2*(2), 1–7. Retrieved March 18, 2006, from http://www.studentaffairs.com/ejournal/ Spring_2001/services.html

Walker, J. M. (1990). Distance education—A model for physical therapy delivery issues. *Journal of Physical Therapy Education, 4*(2), 76–78.

U.S. Department of Education, National Center for Educational Statistics. (2003). *Distance education at degree-granting postsecondary institutions: 2000–2001.* NCES 2003-017 (Tiffany Walts and Laurie Lewis, Project Officer: Bernard Greene). Washington, DC. Retrieved March 18, 2006, from http://nces.ed.gov/pubs2003/2003017.pdf

Chapter 11

A Focus on Older Adults: From Online to CD-ROM

Linda Felver and Catherine Van Son

T his chapter addresses the development of educational innovations by nurse educators involved in the Older Adult Focus Project, directed toward a goal of increasing the ability of nurses to provide care for older adults. As part of that project, we created the Older Adult Focus as a set of materials built into an existing online baccalaureate program for registered nurses (RNs). We then enlarged our scope to develop a stand-alone CD-ROM designed for multiple purposes: to assist nursing students and RNs to increase their abilities in working with older adults and to assist educators who want to infuse older adult content into existing courses or teach it as a separate course. This initial innovation and its subsequent evolution into a second innovation arose in the context of the imbalance between the health care needs of older adults and the availability of nurses educated to work with this population. The development process we used can be adapted to other educational settings and is the focus of this chapter.

The Context

The context in which these innovations arose includes the increasing health needs of older adults, decreasing availability of nurses, the need

This chapter was accepted on April 2, 2006.

for nurses with competencies in caring for older adults in many different health care settings, and the severe health care imbalance in rural areas. Our understanding of this context shaped the development of our innovations.

Increasing Health Care Needs of Older Adults

Older adults (persons aged 65 and over) have complex health care needs due to sensory and other changes of normal aging, decreased physiological reserve capacity, multiple chronic diseases, complicated drug regimens, and multiple psychosocial issues. Older adults comprised 12.4% of the U.S. population in 2000, and this percentage is projected to increase over time (He, Sengupta, Velkoff, DeBarros, & U.S. Census Bureau, 2005; U.S. Census Bureau, 2001). In Oregon, for example, older adults comprised 12.8% of the population in 2000, which was near the national average, and more than 20% of the population is projected to be older than 65 by 2025 (U.S. Census Bureau, 2001; Oregon Health Division, 1999).

As in many parts of the United States, more than 70% of deaths in Oregon are due to cardiovascular disease (heart disease and stroke), cancer, diabetes, and chronic lung disease (Oregon Health Division, 1999). All of these conditions are more prevalent in older adults. These and other chronic conditions, such as arthritis and osteoporosis that are common in older adults, can lead to decreased quality of life and repeated costly hospitalizations. Access to nurses knowledgeable about chronic disease management can improve quality of life and reduce hospitalizations for older adults who have chronic conditions (Kralik, 2005; Quinn et al., 2004). Depression and anxiety are frequently associated with chronic illness. Many older adults have multiple chronic conditions that increase the complexity of their health care needs. Increasing numbers of older adults are becoming caregivers for their spouses; many older adult caregivers have chronic conditions themselves that make caregiving a challenge (Lyons, Stewart, Archbold, Carter, & Perrin, 2004). Nurses need education to prepare them for caring for older adults (Jeffers & Campbell, 2005; Scott-Tilley, Marshall-Gray, Valadez, & Green, 2005).

Decreasing Availability of Nurses

Nursing workforce projections show an acute worsening of the current national nursing shortage in the future, as health care needs escalate and aging nurses retire. By 2020, the United States is estimated to have 400,000 fewer nurses than today—a situation of concern when at the same time baby boomers will be in their 70s and 80s (Hassmiller & Cozine, 2006). The shortage of RNs that exists nationally is also a problem in Oregon. A survey from the Northwest Health Foundation (2001) showed that the mean age of Oregon RNs was 47, which is higher than the national average of 44 years; 60% of the RNs were 45 and older; and 38% were 50 or older. As these nurses retire, projections are for nearly 3,000 fewer RNs available in Oregon in 2010, creating a shortage of more than 20% (Northwest Health Foundation, 2001).

Oregon, similar to other locations, has an increasing need for baccalaureate-prepared nurses who can analyze complex systems, and manage and provide nursing services to individuals, families, groups, and populations (Northwest Health Foundation, 2001). As the population ages and their health care needs increase, older adult nursing competencies are also increasingly necessary to meet the complex needs of older adults.

Need for Nurses With Older Adult Competencies

Older adults receive nursing care in multiple settings. Nurses who work in long-term care work primarily with older adults, who comprise 91% of the nursing home population (U.S. Census Bureau, 2001). However, only 4.5% of persons aged 65 and over live in nursing homes. Therefore, nurses who work in other settings also need older adult nursing competencies (Health Resources and Services Administration, 1995). Home health nurses average 80% older adults in their caseloads. In hospitals, 60% of the patients are 65 or older. Given the ubiquity of older adults in most clinical settings, large numbers of nurses work with older adults. Many of these nurses need to increase their competencies in caring for older adults. Some nursing programs do not provide specific education in older adult nursing. Faculty continue to debate whether gerontological nursing should be a separate course or integrated into the existing curriculum (Wallace, Lange, & Grossman, 2005). Faculty who teach in an integrated format often have not had any education in the care of older adults.

Severe Health Care Imbalance in Rural Areas

The imbalance between health care needs of older adults and the availability of nurses educated to work with them is especially acute in rural areas. Nationally, the 2000 census found that rural areas have a higher proportion of older adults in their total population than urban areas (Economic Research Service, 2004). The distribution of older adults is disproportionately high in rural areas due to outmigration of the young and aging-in-place. In other words, young people are leaving rural areas, but older adults are staying and growing older. In Oregon, for example, although older adults comprise 12.8% of the statewide population, the 2000 U.S. Census showed that the percentage of older adults is 17.6% or more in 12 rural counties and 14.4–17.5% in eight rural counties (U.S. Census Bureau, 2001).

Rural populations are more likely to report poorer health status than their more urban counterparts and are also at risk for health disparities (U.S. Department of Health and Human Services, 2000). Heart disease, cancer, and diabetes rates are higher, and fewer preventive health practices and services are used. All of these disease processes have some modifiable risk factors that could be reduced with adequate numbers of health care practitioners providing preventive services. However, the nursing shortage is most acute in rural areas. For example, although only 20% of Oregon's population is urban, 30% of its RNs work in Oregon's one urban county (Area Health Education Centers Program, 2001). The needs of rural older adults are fast becoming a health care crisis (Economic Research Service, 2004).

Summary of the Context

Nurses are in short supply in many clinical settings that have a high proportion of older adults. Many associate degree nurses who are currently practicing in those settings did not have older adult nursing content in their programs to provide the expertise that they now need with an aging population. In addition, baccalaureate-prepared nurses in many settings also need older adult nursing competencies to serve their patient populations. Many nursing faculty need assistance with teaching students to work with older adults. The nursing shortage is projected to move from severe to crisis proportions by 2010 as the nursing workforce ages and retires. Concurrently, the number of older adults is increasing, and they are living longer and creating increased demand for health care services. Rural areas tend to have proportionately more older adults, a higher proportion of chronic diseases, and fewer nurses. This is the situation that galvanized us into creating the Older Adult Focus and then to modify our set of materials within existing online courses into a stand-alone CD-ROM for wider use.

Available Approaches

Given the context, we examined available approaches to increasing the number of nurses who are knowledgeable regarding working with older adults and determined that they were not sufficient to address the situation. These available approaches included one-time events such as in-service presentations in clinical settings, continuing education workshops, audio broadcasts, and videoconferences; audiovisuals that could be rented or purchased; printed materials such as books and articles in professional journals; and materials available on the Internet. Given the context of rural settings, which are areas of critical need, many of these options are not practical due to distance (e.g., continuing education workshops) or limited local resources (e.g., limited access to professional journals, in print or electronic).

However, we were fortunate that Oregon Health & Science University (OHSU) School of Nursing has a thriving established RN/BS distance learning program. Through this program, nurses are able to earn their BSN without extensive travel to a classroom. They learn from courses delivered via the Internet and CD-ROMs, which is an ideal situation for rural as well as urban settings. The RN/BS program had recently changed from an objective-based curriculum to one that is competency based (Salveson & Cook, 2006). Creating an innovation within this existing program was the most practical way to increase nurses' knowledge about care of older adults, because we could use existing administrative structures and relationships without needing to create our own.

The Older Adult Focus Project

The Older Adult Focus is a set of learning activities that assists students to develop Older Adult Competencies and includes competency evaluations. We developed and implemented these learning activities and competency evaluations through the Older Adult Focus Project, a partnership between the OHSU School of Nursing Gerontological Nursing Specialty Faculty, the OHSU School of Nursing RN/BS program, and The John A. Hartford Center of Geriatric Nursing Excellence at OHSU. The project built the Older Adult Focus option into the existing online curriculum of the OHSU School of Nursing RN/BS program using currently operating distance technology to deliver the program to associate degree-prepared nurses living in rural and other areas of Oregon. In addition to the standard baccalaureate competencies, RNs who complete the Older Adult Focus RN/BS curriculum develop Older Adult Competencies that enable them to provide complex care to older adults in diverse clinical settings. As the Older Adult Focus Project evolved, project personnel created a second innovation: a stand-alone CD-ROM for self-directed learning that provides resources for students, practicing nurses, and faculty. Development of our innovations, which is the focus of this discussion, had four major aspects (as illustrated in Figure 11.1).

Crafting the Nine Older Adult Competencies

Over a period of 11 months, the Gerontological Nursing Specialty Faculty of OHSU School of Nursing developed nine competencies (Older Adult Competencies) with associated components to be demonstrated by Older Adult Focus baccalaureate students. These competencies are presented in Table 11.1. The process of crafting these competencies was an iterative one, with feedback from Gerontological Nursing Specialty faculty, employers, and nurses who work with older adults. Source materials for their development included the 30 recommended baccalaureate competencies for geriatric nursing identified by the American

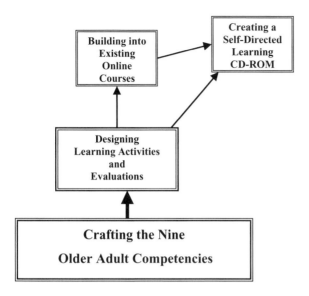

FIGURE 11.1   Model for creating the older adult focus innovations.

Association of Colleges of Nursing and The John A. Hartford Foundation Institute for Geriatric Nursing (2001), materials from the Hartford Institute for Geriatric Nursing at New York University (Mariano, Gould, Mezey, & Fulmer, 1999), and an unpublished document from the Oregon Geriatric Center (1995). Following the model of Lenburg (1999), we revised objectives (pieces of knowledge to learn) from these documents into competencies (specifications of what the nurse does with the knowledge).

Each competency was explicated with multiple components that illustrated its scope. A sample component from each competency is included in Table 11.1. The nine Older Adult Competencies were the foundation on which we built the Older Adult Focus materials, as illustrated in Figure 11.1.

Integrating Older Adult Competencies and Learning Materials

We developed the learning activities and competency evaluations in two phases: First, we built the online materials into the existing courses

TABLE 11.1   The Older Adult Focus Competencies

Older Adult Focus Competency	Example of a Component of the Competency
Awareness: Increase own and others' awareness of attitudes, values, and expectations about aging and their impact on care of older adults and their families.	Implement an activity that increases others' awareness of their attitudes, values, and expectations about aging and their impact on care of older adults and their families.
Communication: Communicate effectively, respectfully, and compassionately with older adults and their families/caregivers.	Use techniques to reduce barriers to communication created by sensory and other physical changes of older adults.
Assessment: Use appropriate assessments for the functional, physical, cognitive, psychological, social, and spiritual status of older adults.	Select assessment tools for areas important to care of older adults (functional status, pressure ulcer risk, mental status, pain, depression, grief, substance abuse, medication history, stages of readiness for change, expressed needs and preferences), based on characteristics of the older adult and the context of care.
Adapting Care: Plan, implement, and evaluate care that is adapted to meet the individual functional, physical, cognitive, psychological, social, and endurance capabilities of older adults.	Plan, implement, and evaluate evidence-based strategies (at a beginning level) to prevent, recognize, and manage geriatric syndromes common to older adults (delirium, dementia, pressure ulcers, polypharmacy, pain, urinary incontinence, sleep disturbance, problems of eating and feeding, falls).
Maximizing Function: Plan, implement, and evaluate care that assists older adults and their families/caregivers to meet personal goals, express preferences, maximize function, maintain desired level of autonomy and independence, and live in their chosen environment.	Assess older adults' living environment and suggest adaptations to optimize person-environment fit, with special awareness of functional, physical, cognitive, psychological, and social changes common in old age.

TABLE 11.1 *(Continued)*

Older Adult Focus Competency	Example of a Component of the Competency
Optimal Aging: Plan, implement, and evaluate care that promotes optimal aging.	Plan and evaluate strategies to promote/maintain physical and mental function and engagement with life in older adults.
Complex Decisions: Guide older adults and their families/caregivers in making complex decisions that arise with aging.	Guide older adults and their families/caregivers to weigh the opportunities and constraints of supportive living arrangements on function and independence.
Organizational Systems: Work effectively within and across organizational systems to promote quality care for older persons.	Facilitate communication as older adults transition between home and different care settings, with a particular focus on the use of technology.
Advocacy: Advocate for health, social, and financial needs of older adults at the policy level.	Work within political, regulatory, and policy-making systems to advocate for resources for older adults and their families who are unable to do this for themselves.

and, second, we developed additional materials for the CD-ROM. The underlying principles we used were the same in both phases.

Designing Learning Activities and Evaluations

While we were designing learning activities to assist in developing the older adult competencies and evaluations of competency development, we applied a standard set of criteria, often in the form of questions.

- Questions guiding development of learning activities:
  - What competency does this activity help develop?
  - Is this activity built on adult learning principles?
  - Have we included guidance for a person using this activity independently?

- Considering all the various learning activities developed for this competency, have we provided options for diverse learning styles?
- Questions guiding development of competency evaluations:
  - Will a person who completes this evaluation really demonstrate components of this competency?
  - Is this evaluation practical or worthwhile doing beyond its evaluative purpose?
  - Are the grading criteria clear enough for a person to use them independently?
  - Considering the options developed for evaluation of this competency, have we provided choices that would appeal to different learning styles?

Focusing on the Competency to be Developed. We designed the learning activities by focusing on the outcome we desired: development of the nine Older Adult Competencies. Each learning activity we created was directed toward assisting a student or practicing nurse to develop a specific component of one of the competencies. No potential learning activity, however intriguing or successfully used in other settings, was included in our materials unless it could be tied directly to a competency. We considered the competencies one at a time and created multiple ways of developing each competency. Although this approach, based on work by Wiggins and McTighe (2001), was a new way of thinking for some of the four faculty who assisted in developing the materials, it soon became the norm for all of our work sessions.

Using Principles of Adult Learning. We incorporated adult learning principles when developing our learning activities (Knowles, Holton, & Swanson, 2005). For example, because adults are independent learners and often approach learning as problem solving, we provided resources to use rather than providing pages of information in a didactic manner. We included alternate learning activities for different clinical settings, so that the learning activities would be seen as having immediate value and have linkage to past experiences. Bearing in mind the context, we supplied resources applicable to both rural and urban settings. For example, one learning activity regarding driving and offered older adults a choice of a rural-focused or an urban-focused journal article to read.

Building in Some Guidance. Because the learning activities we were creating were electronic and commonly would be used in settings without a teacher present, we built guidance into each one. For example, when assigning a journal article, we listed some questions to explore or important areas of focus while reading it. When providing a Web site link, we noted what the focus of the exploration should be or provided a problem to be addressed. When creating PowerPoint presentations, we embedded questions for thought into the screens rather than providing a passive experience. This approach enabled us to create useful learning activities that could be used by individuals working by themselves, as well as those working in groups or with a teacher. The context of the nursing shortage and severe health care needs of older adults in rural areas was an important consideration in our care with providing guidance, because nurses in rural areas often work in isolation.

Providing Options for Diverse Learning Styles. Based on work by Fleming (2001) and Dunn and Dunn (1993) indicating that people have different preferred styles of taking in information, we deliberately created multiple learning activities for each competency that involved diverse modes such as text, pictures, audio clips, video clips, some tactile and kinesthetic experiences, and opportunities to talk with others. This approach was directed vigorously toward the learning activities for the CD-ROM. It required sustained creativity, as well as learning some new technology.

Tying Evaluations to the Competencies. As with the development of learning activities, we kept the desired outcomes (the competencies) as the focus when we designed the evaluations. Each idea for evaluation was scrutinized to determine what components of a specific competency it would allow a learner to demonstrate.

Making the Evaluations Inherently Useful. Rather than evaluate competency development through examinations or formal academic papers, we intentionally designed many of the competency evaluations on the CD-ROM to have usefulness beyond their evaluative purpose. The endproduct might be something that could be used again, such as a patient education brochure adapted for use by older adults, or it might be a way of sharing knowledge about older adults with others, such as providing in-service education for nursing staff with a written reflection on the experience. This approach arose from the principles of adult learning (providing immediate value) and also from the context of increasing health needs of older adults, decreasing availability of nurses, and the need for nurses with older adult competencies in different health care settings. We chose to devise ways that the learners could begin making a difference immediately.

Including the Grading Criteria. We included specific grading criteria with each description of competency evaluation. Our purposes were to let the learners know the expectations, and based on the context of nursing faculty needs, to provide support for other educators who are integrating care of older adults into their courses.

In summary, we used a consistent, deliberative approach to development of learning activities and competency evaluations that was based on educational principles and focused by the societal context for the Older Adult Project.

Building the Older Adult Focus Into Existing Online Courses

Using the aforementioned principles, we built the Older Adult Focus materials into the existing RN/BS curriculum. Noteworthy aspects of this development included creating a map, modifying existing learning activities and evaluations, and establishing an identifier for our online materials.

Creating a Map. The existing RN/BS curriculum had 11 upper division courses into which we needed to incorporate development of the nine older adult competencies without creating a separate course. To accomplish this processes, we needed to map the competencies across the courses. This work was facilitated by the team approach used by the RN/BS program at OHSU (Salveson & Cook, 2006). We met with the entire RN/BS faculty and worked together to map the competencies across the courses, using a grid approach (Table 11.2). The RN/BS curriculum at that time had a standard sequence of courses so we were able to establish in which courses each competency would be developed and demonstrated. After competency demonstration, Older Adult Focus students would be expected to apply the competency in subsequent courses. This process was familiar to most of the faculty, because they had

TABLE 11.2 Partial Grid Showing Relationship of Older Adult Competencies to RN/BS Courses

Older Adult Competencies	Health Assessment	Research	Community Nursing Clinical	Health Policy	Ethics	Reflective Practice Clinical
Awareness	Demo		Apply	Apply	Apply	Apply
Communication	Demo		Apply	Apply	Apply	Apply
Assessment	Demo		Apply		Apply	Apply
Adapting Care	Prep	Prep	Prep			Demo
Maximizing Function	Prep	Prep	Prep	Prep		Demo
Optimal Aging	Prep	Prep	Prep	Prep		Demo
Complex Decisions	Prep	Prep	Prep		Demo	Apply
Organizational Systems	Prep		Demo	Apply	Apply	Apply
Advocacy	Prep		Prep	Demo	Apply	Apply

Note: Prep, competency development; Demo, competency evaluation; Apply, competency use is expected.

created a similar grid for program competencies during development of the RN/BS curriculum (Salveson & Cook, 2006).

Modifying Existing Learning Activities and Evaluations. The RN/BS faculty gave us access to existing course materials for the online courses. We chose one gerontological nursing textbook that Older Adult Focus students could use during all of their courses. Using the principles described in the previous section, we created new learning activities and modified existing ones (as shown in the examples in Table 11.3) to guide students toward development of the older adult competencies.

When building the older adult competency evaluations into each course, our primary approach was to modify existing course evaluations so the students would be able to demonstrate their regular course competencies and the Older Adult Focus competencies simultaneously. For example, the competency demonstration for the health assessment course was a complete nursing assessment with a self-made videotape of the student conducting a physical examination. The students were able to demonstrate their assessment competency (one of the nine older adult competencies) by completing this course assignment with an older adult, including an appropriate screening tool for older adults, and demonstrating the specialized assessment skills they had learned in the Older Adult Focus portion of the course. The students appreciated our practical approach to combining two purposes within one assignment.

Establishing an Identifier. One of the principles of effective online teaching and learning is to organize materials in ways that provide ease of access. Because we were embedding Older Adult Focus materials into online courses in which both regular RN/BS and Older Adult Focus RN/BS students were enrolled, we devised a green-bordered box that became the identifier for Older Adult Focus materials within each online course. Mindful of our societal context, with the need for nurses to be skilled in care of older adults and faculty to improve their knowledge as well, we decided to make the Older Adult Focus materials visible to all students in the online courses. The success of this approach was borne out by positive comments from RN/BS students who used our green boxes even though they were not Older Adult Focus students. In addition, one of the course faculty was so pleased with a major portion of the Older Adult Focus learning activities developed for her course

TABLE 11.3   Examples of Older Adult Focus Adaptations in an Existing Health Assessment Course

Topic	Existing Online Course	Older Adult Focus
Head and Neck Examination	Find one Web site or journal article discussing examination of the head and neck (e.g., finding nits and lice, effectively palpating the thyroid gland, lymph node examination). Share what you have learned with your classmates by posting the reference and describing the contents.	Find one Web site or journal article discussing assessment, risk factors and referrals related to dysphagia (swallowing disorder), xerostomia (dry mouth), oral candidiasis (thrush), or other oral disorders in older adults. Share what you have learned with your classmates by posting the reference and describing the contents.
Musculoskeletal Examination	One method of assessing hip function is the Stahli examination (Children's Hospital, Seattle, Washington). This screening tool is included in the discussion area. Try it on another adult and report your findings.	The "Get Up and Go Test" is an assessment that should be conducted as part of a routine evaluation when working with older persons. Its purpose is to detect those at risk for falling and to identify those who need further evaluation. Try the "Get Up and Go Test" on an older adult. You will find this screening tool described in the Older Adult discussion area. Report your findings.

that, with our permission, she incorporated them into the course for all students in future terms.

While we were building the Older Adult Focus into the existing courses and had admitted more than 50 students into the Older Adult Focus Project, rapid changes occurred, including curriculum revision in the RN/BS program, change from one admission cycle per year to two, and availability of weekend intensive courses that students could choose as an alternative to online courses. Faculty in other courses had heard about our materials and were asking to use them. In addition, we knew that our grant funding was time-limited and, ever mindful of our societal context, we wanted to sustain the Older Adult Focus in the future. For these reasons, we decided to create an Older Adult Focus CD-ROM that could be used separately from existing courses or in conjunction with them and could also be used as a resource by faculty.

Creating an Older Adult Focus CD-ROM for Self-Directed Learning

The Older Adult Focus CD-ROM is a compilation of educational materials to facilitate the development and demonstration of the nine Older Adult Competencies. It can be used for the following purposes:

- as a self-directed study resource for nursing students or RNs,
- as individual learning activities for faculty to use in any course that they teach,
- as content to be integrated into a curriculum, or
- as the basis for a stand-alone gerontological nursing course.

For each of the nine Older Adult Competencies, the CD-ROM includes a menu of learning activities to assist with competency development and a choice of competency evaluations (with grading criteria) for demonstrating the competency. Aspects of creating the CD-ROM that will be discussed here include the following:

- developing a template,
- maintaining consistency and variety,
- planning for longevity,
- mastering technological challenges, and
- pilot testing.

Developing a Template. To provide consistency and usability, we designed a template that we could use for each module on the CD-ROM. A major consideration was the purpose of our CD-ROM. Because we intended it to be used as a resource disc rather than as an online course, we created our template accordingly. We created the materials for each competency as a separate web of files, resolved navigational issues within and between competencies, and used color coding and graphics to orient the users to their location within the CD-ROM. In an attempt to model what we were teaching, we incorporated the color contrast and font aspects that are most effective for aging eyes. At all times, we kept in mind the isolated learner—a person who might be using the CD-ROM with no external support or guidance.

Maintaining Consistency and Variety. Although we were able to reuse many of the materials we had developed for the online Older Adult Focus, creating a CD-ROM for self-directed learning opened up many new possibilities. We were no longer constrained by pre-existing courses into which we needed to fit. Using the principles described previously, we designed a large menu of learning activities for each competency so that learners have the opportunity to select those activities that best suit their learning style, resources, and clinical setting (Billings, Connors, & Skiba, 2001). Similarly, we provided alternative ways of evaluating each competency. We also attended to consistency with regard to aspects such as terminology, level of difficulty, and format of instructions, while intentionally creating variety in the types of learning activities and choices of competency demonstrations. In other words, we focused on the details while simultaneously considering the complete scope of the product we were creating.

Planning for Longevity. Realizing that revision of a CD-ROM is more difficult and costly than revision of materials in an online course, we were attentive to selecting materials that we expected to be stable over time. For example, when we directed the learners to an external resource, we linked to the top level of a Web site, rather than to an inner page, so that the link would still function after any reorganization of the Web site. In addition, we provided key words to assist in finding a similar site in case of Web site disappearance.

Mastering Technological Challenges. Because one of us (L. F.) had substantial prior experience with developing and maintaining course websites with multiple webs of HTML documents, we were able to create the CD-ROM at a relatively low cost by doing most of the technical work ourselves. Our concern for providing learning activities for multiple learning styles mandated the learning of technology for creating and linking such items as audio clips, video clips, and crossword puzzles that can be completed electronically. Learning and incorporating the technological aspects of creating an accessible CD-ROM for persons with low vision or hearing deficit was another important task. The major challenge with the technology was time, because the same person who was responsible for the technological aspects was also the leader of the team for pedagogical aspects of the project.

Pilot Testing. We pilot tested portions of our materials for the CD-ROM by posting an extensive web within one of the online courses, with permission from the course faculty. Older Adult Focus students in the course that term were enthusiastic, and the course faculty requested the materials be available again the next time the course was taught. We sent trial versions of several competencies to numerous faculty for comment. In addition, we sent full versions of some of the competency materials on CD-ROM to several students who provided specific positive comments on some of the navigational features, as well as the learning activities. One student successfully developed and demonstrated successfully two of the competencies using this test CD-ROM, which showed us that our approach was feasible. The outcome of our pilot testing was consistent with research by Maag (2004) and Tsai et al. (2004), which demonstrated effectiveness of multimedia approaches to learning.

Application to Other Settings

Many of the processes we used during development of our innovations can be used in other settings where groups are working on desired outcomes, creating learning activities and evaluations for competency-based learning, planning to build specialty content into general courses, or wishing to develop a CD-ROM for self-directed learning.

Suggestions for Drafting Desired Outcome Statements

We shall highlight here two aspects of the process we used to craft the nine Older Adult Competencies and their components that could be used successfully in other institutions.

Brainstorm Before Using Existing Materials and Networks. After an initial brainstorming session with the Gerontological Nursing Specialty Faculty, one of us (L. F.) wrote a first draft of the competencies that integrated the ideas from the meeting and materials from the source documents described earlier (the American Association of College of Nurses and The John A. Hartford Foundation Institute for Geriatric Nursing, 2001; Mariano et al., 1999). This process facilitated creative thinking, provided an opportunity for us to use our own expertise, and then enabled us to validate and extend our own ideas with nationally recognized sources.

In addition, our ability to tie into existing academic-practice linkages was invaluable. When we wanted feedback from employers and nurses who work with older adults, we asked the community partners of The John A. Hartford Center of Geriatric Nursing Excellence at OHSU, who gave useful feedback within our suggested time frame. Using this existing network was efficient and effective.

Use an Iterative Process. We found that an iterative process was ideal for developing a set of competencies. Because we established the expectation at the beginning, the Gerontological Nursing Specialty Faculty knew that the initial drafts would receive feedback, undergo revision, and improve until all persons involved were satisfied. This expectation kept each of us from premature attachment to our own ideas and enabled 17 faculty to come to agreement in a remarkable teamwork fashion.

Suggestions for Designing Competency-Based Learning Materials

The approach we used for designing learning activities and competency evaluations is applicable to any setting in which people are planning teaching and learning.

Focus on Desired Outcomes. If we begin driving without knowing our destination, we have little chance of arriving there. By analogy, we need to decide where we want the learners to be (i.e., desired outcomes or competencies) and then design learning activities to help them move in that direction (Wiggins & McTighe, 1998). We highly recommend use of the questions that we presented earlier in this chapter to guide development of learning activities and competency evaluations.

Remember Context in Which Learning Will Occur. The context in which the Older Adult Focus was developed led us to apply principles of adult learning; provide guidance with our learning activities for individuals who might use them in isolation; develop materials for persons with different learning styles; create competency evaluations that had inherent usefulness beyond their evaluative purpose; and provide detailed grading criteria to support both students and faculty. Although these enhancements would most likely be useful in any setting, attending to the context can assist with generating creative and effective innovations.

Suggestions for Building a Specialty Focus Into Existing Courses

The processes we used to build the Older Adult Focus into the RN/BS curriculum can be used in any setting where the plan is to build a specialty focus into existing courses.

Create an Overall Map. Mapping the desired outcomes of a specialty focus against the existing courses is an excellent way to provide an overall plan that facilitates the parts fitting into the whole without duplication, redundancies, or major omissions. If two sets of faculty are involved, as with Older Adult Focus faculty and the regular RN/BS faculty, having them create such a map together is beneficial in building teamwork and generating commitment toward a common goal.

Be Mindful of Student Workload. A concern of many faculty in the RN/BS program, and of Older Adult Focus faculty as well, was not overloading students with additional work. We addressed that concern by creative modification of existing learning activities and evaluations to include older adults. In many cases, substituting an older adult as the client of focus worked well. In other cases, we added older adult learning activities in ways that kept the flavor of a course but expanded its scope. Faculty and students responded well to these approaches, which are useful to consider when building specialty content into general courses.

Use Identifiers for Specialty Content and Make It Accessible. Providing a mechanism such as our separate green boxes for Older Adult Focus students is a useful approach to avoid confusion in a course that has both general and specialty students. As described previously, the general students and course faculty also benefited from this approach. In addition, such an approach could be used beneficially when pilot-testing material that will eventually be integrated fully into a course.

Suggestions for Creating a CD-ROM for Self-Directed Learning

Our previous discussion of processes involved in creating a CD-ROM contains many applications for use by anyone who plans a similar project. We shall summarize briefly here.

Remember the Isolated User. A key approach to developing a CD-ROM for self-directed learning is to remember the isolated user who will interface with the CD-ROM alone at home. This consideration will guide effective creation of a template that provides consistent location of materials, ease of navigation, and orientation to location within the file structure. The concept of the isolated learner also provides a reminder to be consistent with terminology and precisely clear with instructions, as well as to build in some variety and other ways to maintain motivation. Pilot testing with the intended users is important before finalizing the CD-ROM, to see if it indeed meets the needs of the isolated user.

Plan for Technological Aspects in Advance. The complexity of the technology involved in creating a CD-ROM depends in part on the various types of media that will be incorporated and the context in which it will be used. During the planning period, attention to types of media and issues—such as access for persons with low vision and hearing deficits, cost, and time—will be beneficial.

Conclusion

We live in an environment of rapid change, increasing technology, and multiple demands on our time—an environment in which the complex health care needs of older adults are increasing and the availability of nurses educated to provide care to those older adults is decreasing. In this context, we developed innovations for both online learning and self-directed learning from a CD-ROM to help meet the educational needs of nursing faculty, students, and practicing nurses who work with older adults.

Acknowledgment

The Older Adult Focus Project was supported by a grant from the Health Resources and Services Administration, Department of Health and Human Services.

REFERENCES

American Association of Colleges of Nursing (AACN) and The John A. Hartford Foundation Institute for Geriatric Nursing. (2001). *Older adults: Recommended baccalaureate competencies and curricular guidelines for geriatric nursing care.* Washington, DC: AACN.

Area Health Education Centers Program. (2001). *Oregon health workforce project: Registered nurse profile, 2000.* Portland, OR: OHSU.

Billings, D. M., Connors, H. R., & Skiba, D. J. (2001). Benchmarking best practices in web-based nursing courses. *Advances in Nursing Science, 23,* 41–52.

Dunn, R., & Dunn, K. (1993). *Teaching secondary students through their individual learning styles.* Needham Heights, MA: Allyn and Bacon.

Economic Research Service (ERS). (2004). *Rural population and migration: Rural older population.* Retrieved March 28, 2006, from http://www.ers.usda.gov/briefing/population/older/

Fleming, N. (2001). *Teaching and learning styles: VARK strategies.* Christchurch, NZ: Author.

Hassmiller, S., & Cozine, M. (2006). Addressing the nursing shortage to improve the quality of patient care: Efforts of the RWJF and selected funders around the nation to fix this problem in today's hospitals. *Health Affairs, 25,* 268–274.

He, W., Sengupta, M., Velkoff, V. A., DeBarros, K., & U.S. Census Bureau. (2005). *65+ in the United States, 2005* (Current Population Reports P23-209). Washington, DC: U.S. Government Printing Office.

Health Resources and Services Administration. (1995). *A national agenda for geriatric education: White papers*, Vol. 1. Washington, DC: U.S. Department of Health and Human Services.

Jeffers, B. R., & Campbell, S. L. (2005). Preparing to care for older adults: Engaging college constituents. *Journal of Nursing Education, 44*, 280–282.

Knowles, M. S., Holton, E. F., & Swanson, R. A. (Eds.). (2005). *The adult learner: The definitive classic in adult education and human resource development* (6th ed.). Burlington: Elsevier.

Kralik, D. (2005). How did patients with comorbidities who required an acute hospital stay perceive the quality of acute care services? *Evidence-based Nursing, 8*, 30–33.

Lenburg, C. (1999, September 30). The framework, concepts and methods of the competency outcomes and performance assessment (COPA) model. *Online Journal of Issues in Nursing*. Retrieved March, 22, 2000, from http://www.nursingworld.org/ojin/topic10/tpc10_2.htm

Lyons, K. S., Stewart, B. J., Archbold, P. G., Carter, J. H., & Perrin, N. A. (2004). Pessimism and optimism as early warning signs for compromised health for caregivers of patients with Parkinson's disease. *Nursing Research, 63*, 354–362.

Maag, M. (2004). The effectiveness of an interactive multimedia learning tool on nursing students' math knowledge and self-efficacy. *CIN: Computers, Informatics, Nursing, 22*, 26–33.

Mariano, C., Gould, E., Mezey, M., & Fulmer, T. (Eds.). (1999). *Best nursing practices in care for older adults: Incorporating essential gerontologic content into baccalaureate nursing education* (2nd ed.). New York: Hartford Institute for Geriatric Nursing, New York University.

Northwest Health Foundation. (2001). *Oregon's nursing shortage: A public health crisis in the making*. Portland, OR: Author.

Oregon Geriatric Education Center. (1995). *Knowledge, skills, and abilities needed to work with older people*. Unpublished paper.

Oregon Health Division. (1999). *Keeping Oregonians healthy: An assessment of leading causes of death and related behaviors in Oregon*. Portland, OR: Author.

Quinn, M. E., Berding, C., Daniels, E., Gerlach, M. J., Harris, K., Nugent, K., et al. (2004). Shifting paradigms: Teaching gerontological nursing from a new perspective. *Journal of Gerontological Nursing, 30*, 21–27.

Salveson, C., & Cook, L. R. (2006). Transforming RN/BS distance education: Competency-based approach using course CD-ROMs. *Annual Review of Nursing Education, 4*, 103–127.

Scott-Tilley, D., Marshall-Gray, P., Valadez, A., & Green, A. (2005). Integrating long-term care concepts into baccalaureate nursing education: the road to quality geriatric healthcare. *Journal of Nursing Education, 44*, 286–290.

Tsai, S. L., Tsai, W. W., Chai, S. K., Sung, W. H., Doong, J. L., & Fung, C. P. (2004). Evaluation of computer-assisted multimedia instruction in intravenous injection. *International Journal of Nursing Studies, 41*, 191–198.

U.S. Census Bureau. (2001). *The 65 years and over population: 2000, Census 2000 Brief*, C2KBR/01-10. Washington, DC: Author.

U.S. Department of Health and Human Services. (2000). *Healthy people 2010* (Conference ed.). Washington, DC: Author.

Wallace, M., Lange, J., & Grossman, S. (2005). Isolation followed by integration: A model for development of a separate geriatric course. *Journal of Nursing Education, 44*, 253–256.

Wiggins, G., & McTighe, J. (2001). *Understanding by design*. Upper Saddle River, NJ: Merrill Prentice-Hall.

Chapter 12

Enriching Student Learning and Enhancing Teaching Through a Course Management System

Linda M. Goodfellow

Several years ago, the faculty at Duquesne University School of Nursing adopted a course management system (CMS) to manage all courses taught in the School of Nursing. A CMS is a Web-based "frame" through which faculty can communicate with students, distribute information, and facilitate the exchange of ideas, information, and resources. A CMS offers students easy and immediate access to grades; information about the instructor, office hours, phone contact, and e-mail address; discussion forums and chats; course materials, assignments, resources, announcements, and a calendar of events; and other information.

The purpose of this chapter is to describe how the use of an educational technology tool—such as a CMS—can enrich student learning and enhance teaching. The chapter discusses what prompted faculty to adopt a CMS, reviews the literature on CMSs, describes innovative ways in which a CMS is used in both the traditional and virtual classroom, examines the pros and cons of using a CMS, and discusses the significant role a CMS can play in nursing education.

This chapter was accepted on Februrary 1, 2006.

What Prompted Faculty to Adopt a Course Management System

During the late 1990s, the first completely online PhD program in nursing was offered at Duquesne University School of Nursing via a CMS called First Class©. Shortly thereafter, all courses in the Graduate Master's Program were also delivered online. By the year 2000, Duquesne University purchased the site license for a CMS called Blackboard® (http://www.blackboard.com). Since then, all online courses have been offered on Blackboard. Faculty, regardless of whether they taught in the doctoral or master's program, attended an 8-hour orientation and completed the Blackboard CMS tutorial.

The advantages of using a CMS for all levels of nursing education seemed obvious. Several faculty teaching undergraduate courses in the traditional classroom setting began requesting course sites, uploading their course materials, and requiring students to access the course site on a regular basis to check announcements. This proved to be cost effective as the volume of paper used to print course profiles, syllabi, and class schedules was drastically reduced. Also, it was an easy, effective way of communicating to large groups of students by sending e-mail to all users or select users, such as specific clinical groups. Posting announcements on the homepage of the course site was used to remind students of due dates, class events, and other activities.

Before long, the course site was used to post case studies and handouts for class, including PowerPoint presentations, which students printed out to facilitate note taking during lecture. Eventually, computer-generated, non-graded quizzes that helped students prepare for their course examinations were uploaded to the CMS. Students could access and take the quizzes whenever they wanted, check their answers, and receive feedback. In addition, students had immediate access to their examination or course project grades once faculty entered grades into the CMS grade book.

Because the School of Nursing had already adopted Blackboard to deliver online courses in the master's and doctoral programs and several faculty members were using it to manage their undergraduate courses, it seemed only natural to require a CMS for all courses offered in the School of Nursing. Those who had never used a CMS were enticed by its appeal and encouraged to consider its use in their own courses.

Background

Much has been reported about distance learning and online education (Baldwin & Burns, 2004; Bernard et al., 2004; Brownson, 2005; Goodfellow, 2002; Hyde & Murray, 2005; Kozlowshi, 2004; Parker, Riza, Tierney, & Barrett, 2005; Patton, Fedorka, & Pavlovich, 2004; Phillips, 2005; Stella & Gnanam, 2004). However, little has been written about the platform in which distance learning courses are offered. In particular, the use of a CMS to enhance learning in traditional, classroom-taught courses has received limited attention in the literature (Neville, 2003).

Stair and Waltz (2004) compared a variety of the most popular courseware management systems, including Blackboard, Web CT, NiceNet, Angel, and Open Source. Cost, learning curve, and overall strengths/weaknesses of delivering online instruction were identified as key factors in determining the selection of a CMS. Blackboard (http://www.blackboard.net) and Web CT (http://www.webct.com) are the most frequently used CMSs, are user-friendly, and offer the most features and flexibility. Both Blackboard and Web CT are costly, whereas NiceNet, Angel, and Open Source are free (Stair & Waltz). In October 2005, Blackboard and Web CT announced their plans to merge. There are also several other courseware management systems available, such as Convene, eCollege.com, Intralearn, and Symposium. An in-depth comparison of online courseware management systems can be found at http://www.marshall.edu/it/cit/Webct/compare.

Innovative Ways to Use a Course Management System

In this section, innovative ways to enrich student learning and enhance teaching through the use of a CMS are discussed for courses taught in the traditional and virtual classroom settings. Specific examples are provided to illustrate how a CMS can be used to teach students at different levels of nursing education.

Using a Course Management System in the Traditional Classroom Setting

A CMS is generally used in the traditional classroom setting to manage course information and course materials, post announcements and grades, and send e-mails to a large group of students at one time. In a nursing research course taught at the undergraduate level, a CMS was used to enhance student learning through the use of cooperative learning strategies.

As a proponent of cooperative learning strategies, I used these strategies to teach an undergraduate nursing research course in the traditional classroom setting without Web enhancement (Goodfellow, 1995) and also to teach an online nursing research course to registered nurses completing their baccalaureate in nursing degree (Goodfellow, 2002). Cooperative learning strategies promote active learning through discussion and sharing of information. In addition, students take responsibility for each other's learning (Stiles, 2006).

Based on previous experiences, I asked the undergraduate nursing students to self-select their formal cooperative learning groups. Then, on Blackboard CMS, I entered the students' names and created their groups, each consisting of three to five students. Controls were set so that only those students belonging to that particular group and the instructor could access their work. I promised the students I would not enter their group unless invited. Controls were also set so that students could send group e-mail, exchange files, use the discussion board, and conduct live chats in the virtual classroom as shown in Figure 12.1.

Class assignments were posted under assignments on the CMS. Students completed a total of four assignments online in their formal cooperative learning groups at either a mutually agreed on time or asynchronously. Once the assignment was complete, one student took responsibility to post it to my digital drop box for me to review, grade, and return to the group's digital drop box.

Students were also required to work on their course project in their cooperative learning groups. Guidelines were posted under course materials on the CMS. The course project consisted of students developing an experimental or quasi-experimental design based on their personal observations from a variety of clinical settings and from gaps identified in the nursing literature. Once students identified a problem or intervention that needed further study, they selected an appropriate population, developed research questions and hypotheses to guide the study, reviewed the literature, and developed the methodology.

Students worked on the project throughout the semester. They were encouraged to do their work on the CMS, avoiding the need to schedule a specific meeting time and yet allowing all group members access to

📖 Manage Groups

👥 **Alice, Kristen, Lisa, Karen, & Emily**   (Modify)
                                                              (Remove)

   🖳Group File Exchange 🗗Group Discussion Board 🖳Group Virtual
   Classroom ✉Group Email
👥 **Amy, Heidy, Regina, Jason, & Kelly**   (Modify)
                                                              (Remove)

   🖳Group File Exchange 🗗Group Discussion Board 🖳Group Virtual
   Classroom ✉Group Email
👥 **Brandi, Ashley & Susan**   (Modify)
                                                              (Remove)

   🖳Group File Exchange 🗗Group Discussion Board 🖳Group Virtual
   Classroom ✉Group Email
👥 **Christine, Luanne, Joan, Elizabeth, & Linda**   (Modify)
                                                              (Remove)

   🖳Group File Exchange 🗗Group Discussion Board 🖳Group Virtual
   Classroom ✉Group Email
👥 **Jackie, John, Roberta, & Julie**   (Modify)
                                                              (Remove)

   🖳Group File Exchange 🗗Group Discussion Board 🖳Group Virtual
   Classroom ✉Group Email
👥 **Hope, Megan, & Carie**   (Modify)
                                                              (Remove)

   🖳Group File Exchange 🗗Group Discussion Board 🖳Group Virtual
   Classroom ✉Group Email

FIGURE 12.1   Controls set for the cooperative learning groups in an undergraduate nursing research course created on Blackboard®

their work at any time, day or night. Most groups expected each group member to contribute to the project on a weekly basis. Their efforts were summarized and presented as a PowerPoint presentation to the entire class at the end of the semester.

Prior to the use of the CMS in the traditional classroom setting, students were required to summarize their research efforts in a poster presentation (Goodfellow, 1995). This required them to buy poster board and other supplies to create the poster, meet at a designated time to plan the poster, and then meet to put the poster together.

Also, students were required to post their PowerPoint presentations on the discussion board for students in the other cooperative learning groups to view, critique, and offer suggestions. This made my role easier because I was able to evaluate the students' presentations online or after downloading to my hard drive as opposed to evaluating the students' group projects on the floor of my office surrounded by 10 to15 posters.

My comments and feedback were posted on the CMS and also sent to the group members via e-mail.

The use of cooperative learning strategies in Web-enhanced traditional courses promotes discovery and stimulates students to share knowledge. In addition, students learn the importance of collaboration and develop leadership, decision-making, and conflict-management skills. Communication skills, albeit electronic, are greatly enhanced and general computer technology skills are increased.

Using a Course Management System in the Virtual Classroom Setting

A CMS is essential when a course is taught online. It is important that the course site is well-organized, easy to navigate, and user-friendly. A well-prepared course syllabus should be posted that identifies and clearly delineates the role the online environment will play in the course.

Using a Course Management System in Clinical and Role Practicum Courses

Offering a Master's clinical or role practicum course online can be a challenge. Students are expected to identify a master's- or doctoral-prepared clinician or educator near to where they live and set up the practicum based on their individual needs. Content of the individualized practicum is planned by the student, faculty, and preceptor in accordance with course objectives, the student's previous experiences and professional goals, and the resources of the agency in which the student is placed.

Learning contracts between student and preceptor are developed, preceptors sign a preceptor agreement form, mutually agreed on contracts between the school of nursing and the agency or institution identified by the student are signed, and students show evidence of health and agency requirements. In addition, preceptors generally want to review the course objectives and need to have access to student evaluation forms. Communication between the student, preceptor, and faculty member is critical.

A CMS can help facilitate this process and make life much easier for the student, preceptor, and faculty member. Templates for learning contracts, preceptor agreement forms, and course objectives can be made accessible to the preceptors by simply providing them access as a guest to the course site. If the preceptor does not want access to the course site, the student can e-mail course information in the form of an attachment or print out the course information and hand deliver it to the preceptor.

Another challenge in an online practicum course is keeping the students grounded in their role. In the typical education role practicum, students meet face-to-face with each other and their teacher in a classroom setting on a regular basis. There, specific topics to the role of an educator are discussed and students can share their experiences.

In an online practicum course, students may live in different parts of the world and may feel disconnected to other students and the faculty member if frequent communication is not offered. The discussion board on Blackboard CMS can help keep students grounded during their role practicum course. A CMS provides the platform by which students can share their experiences and specific topics can be discussed. This creates an environment conducive to learning and helps students remain grounded during a role practicum.

One forum frequently created is called "Share Your Experience." Students are expected to post their experiences on a weekly basis. Similar to a reflective journal, students analyze each others' experiences, dialogue, and engage in active learning.

Other forums are created to discuss specific topics related to nursing education as shown in Table 12.1. A scenario or description of the topic is provided followed by a list of focus questions that students address over a specific time period. Students are expected to engage in a meaningful discussion centered on the focus questions. Table 12.2 provides an example of focus questions used for a specific discussion. A certain degree of latitude is necessary for brainstorming and creative thinking. A specific topic forum is usually kept opened for about 2 weeks, thus giving the students plenty of time to participate. Some forums, however, take on a life of their own, with one topic leading to another throughout the semester. In cases like this, I do not close the forum, but rather encourage students to continue with the discussion.

Using a Course Management System in a Research Seminar Course

I also create several different forums on the discussion board for doctoral students enrolled in a research seminar. This is the last core course

TABLE 12.1   Topics Discussed in a Nursing Education Role Practicum

Role Issues in Nursing Education
Academic Freedom and Tenure
Faculty Practice
Bridging the Gap Between Nursing Education and Nursing Practice
Nurse Educator Career Development
The Curriculum Revolution
Theoretical Bases for the Practice of Nursing Education
Ethical Issues in Nursing Education

Note. Each topic is accompanied by specific focus questions that are posted as a forum for discussion as seen in Table 12.2.

students take in the doctoral program and an appropriate course to teach online because every assignment and topic for discussion has an Internet component associated with it. This is a "nuts and bolts course" of doctoral education because the topics for discussion, as illustrated in Figure 12.2, are all necessary to complete the dissertation successfully. Each topic is accompanied by a set of focus questions that students are expected to answer and discuss during a specific time period. Table 12.3 provides an example of the focus questions developed for discussion related to institutional review boards. For each assignment, students are expected to critique each other's work, offer suggestions, and encourage and support each other.

TABLE 12.2   Example of Focus Questions for Class Discussion in the Nursing Education Role Practicum Course

Over the next 2 weeks I would like you to participate in a discussion related to your role as a nurse educator. Each of you has planned this role practicum to meet the course objectives and your own learning needs. Consequently, your experiences are similar yet differ from others in your class. I anticipate a lively discussion since your past and current experiences in nursing education are so diverse. Please address the following:

1. What is your current role as a nurse educator?
2. What does it mean to be a nurse educator?
3. Will your role change after graduation? If so, how?
4. How will you bridge the nurse educator role with nursing practice?

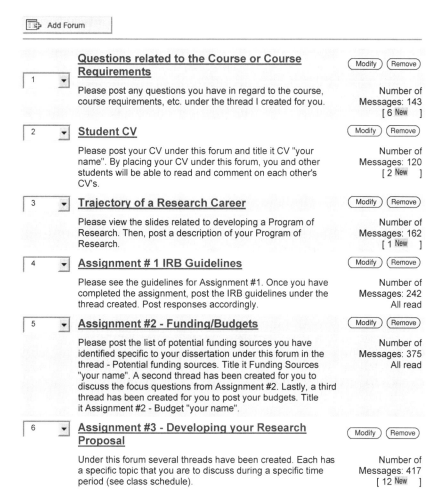

FIGURE 12.2   Forums created on the discussion board for student participation in a research seminar course offered to doctoral students via Blackboard®. CV, curriculum vitae; IRB, institutional review board.

TABLE 12.3   Example of Focus Questions Developed for Discussion in the Research Seminar

Once you have posted the IRB guidelines from the institution or agency you anticipate using for dissertation study and have read your classmates postings, use this message area to post comments. You can use your word processing program to write and save your comments, then copy and paste to this message area. You will not be able to print or change your comments once they are posted in this message area. Issues to consider while you are browsing through different IRB guidelines:

1. What criteria do IRBs use to determine whether the proposed research is ethical or not?
2. Although IRB guidelines may differ from one institution or agency and another, what underlying principles are similar? How do the protocols differ?
3. Under what category will your dissertation study fall? Full-board review, Expedited, or Exempt? Why?
4. Determine the Risk/Benefit ratio for your study. All studies involve some risk, but the risk may be minimal. How does one define minimal risk? Will your study be one of minimal risk?
5. In what ways do the requirements in regard to ethical issues differ from IRB to IRB?
6. Does your IRB offer an example of a consent form? Offer specific guidelines about the the consent form? This may be a good time to begin developing the informed consent related to your dissertation topic or begin thinking (jot down or tape these thoughts) about how you will incorporate the ethical principles underlying the Belmont Report into your research proposal and consent forms.

IRB, institution review board.

Pros and Cons of a Course Management System

Although there are many advantages to using a CMS in both the traditional and virtual classroom settings, the disadvantages must also be considered prior to adopting a CMS. This section addresses the advantages and disadvantages of using a CMS.

Advantages

The advantages of using a CMS far outweigh the disadvantages. Convenience for both students and faculty is the most obvious advantage. For those students living in rural areas or other countries, a CMS provides them with the platform by which they can take courses without leaving their home, providing they have access to a computer and an Internet Service Provider. If the course is conducted in the asynchronous format, different time zones are not a problem because students work on their own time schedule.

Regardless of whether the course is taught in the traditional classroom or online, a CMS permits students to work on group projects, take examinations or quizzes, engage in discussion, and communicate to others, all on their own time. Faculty members have immediate access to the student's work, and can critique and support the student's ideas in a timely manner without carrying assignments home to correct.

Because the course information and materials are all in one place, students can access and read the same information. If a printed document is lost, another can easily be replaced. With the click of a mouse, students have access to specific course information, such as announcements, course profiles, course materials, faculty and student information, assignments, required readings, and external resources. Posting announcements can free class time previously used for updates and reminders. In addition, communication is enhanced via the discussion board, live chats, and e-mail to single or group users. Completed assignments can be posted to the instructor's digital drop box, and PowerPoint presentations can be attached to the discussion board for everyone to view. In addition, there is always an electronic record of live chats and group discussions.

A CMS also fosters active learning and independent learning skills. Assignments and group discussions promote critical thinking skills and encourage peer review. Although the impetus for learning is on the individual student, students share information and knowledge with each other, learn how to work in groups, and support each other's learning. These types of activities promote close student relationships and lifelong professional and personal friendships.

As previously described, the impetus for learning in online education is placed on the student. However, learning can be enhanced by the use of a discussion board via a CMS. Focus questions that stimulate critical thinking and problem solving help create an atmosphere conducive to learning. In addition, students not only learn how to critique each other's work, but also learn to do it in an appropriate way. Students share information, knowledge, and Internet resources. Students engage in meaningful discussions that further promote active learning behaviors, enthusiasm, and a competitive spirit.

Lastly, a CMS promotes skills in computer technology. Students at all levels of nursing education must learn computer skills. At the very least, students learn to send and receive e-mail as well as to attach, send, and open documents from email or Internet sites. In addition, they develop skills by which they can research topics using Internet resources and learn to use Internet library databases.

Disadvantages

Regardless of whether a course site is created for a traditional or an online class, the start-up time is extensive. For a faculty member who is not comfortable with computer technology, this start-up time is grueling. Time must be allotted for training and developing the course site and the course itself. A different mind-set is also necessary as the faculty member begins to develop strategies other than lecture to teach the class. Focus questions for discussion of specific topics on the discussion board must be developed.

All course information, materials, assignments, and guidelines must be prepared and then uploaded onto the CMS course site. It is imperative that the directions and guidelines for each assignment or course project are clearly stated. I have found it helpful to include a forum entitled "Questions" on the discussion board so that students can ask questions about the course, assignments, or projects. Links to Internet resources must be established. Course settings need to be set so that students not only have access to the course site, but also can e-mail each other, exchange files, work in groups, and post attachments or comments on the discussion board.

Both students and faculty who plan to work from home on their course site need to consider either a DSL or Broadband Internet connection. A dial-up connection can be used, but it will be much slower to access and download or upload course materials. Computer requirements are important considerations that will influence the overall experience for both students and faculty. Thus, it is important that students are aware of the minimal computer requirements necessary to access and use online course materials. These are posted on Duquesne University School of Nursing graduate Web site (http://www.nursing.duq.edu/gradOnlTech.html) so that students can view prior to applying for entry into any of the online programs offered.

Training and development of course materials can be time consuming and for those who are not comfortable with computer technology, somewhat frustrating. It is imperative that the University has an infrastructure in place that is supportive, offers training and tutorials, and is available when help is needed. In addition, faculty development sessions should be offered so that new strategies and methods of teaching in the virtual classroom can be learned.

Role of a Course Management System in Nursing Education

Thanks to recent technological advances and Internet capabilities, the possibilities for the use of a CMS are endless. A CMS can be a powerful technological tool for the nurse educator. It can be used to promote independent and group learning, active participation, critical thinking, communication skills, and computer skills. Nurse educators can create a course site that is ideal for the type of content that will be taught. Visual, textual, and auditory activities can be developed to enhance student learning. Invaluable Internet resources can be linked to the course site to supplement required readings and assignments. Regardless of whether a course is taught in the traditional or virtual classroom, a CMS can enrich student learning and enhance teaching.

REFERENCES

Baldwin, K. M., & Burns, P. G. (2004). Development and implementation of an online CNS program. *Clinical Nurse Specialist*, *18*, 248–254.

Bernard, R. M., Abrami, P. C., Lou, Y., Borokhovski, E., Wade, A., Wozney, L., et al. (2004). How does distance education compare with classroom instruction? A meta-analysis of the empirical literature. *Review of Educational Research*, *74*, 379–439.

Brownson, K. (2005). College on the Internet. *Health Care Manager*, *24*(4), 350–355.

Goodfellow, L. M. (1995). Cooperative learning strategies: An effective method of teaching nursing research. *Nurse Educator*, *20*(4), 26–29.

Goodfellow, L. M. (2002). Tips and strategies used to teach an on-line nursing research course. *Nurse Educator*, *27*, 1, 8.

Hyde, A., & Murray, M. (2005). Nurses' experiences of distance education programs. *Journal of Advanced Nursing*, *49*, 87–95.

Kozlowshi, D. (2004). Factors for consideration in the development and implementation of an online RN-BSN course: Faculty and student perceptions. *CIN: Computers, Informatics, Nursing, 22*(1), 34–43.

Neville, M. W. (2003). Blackboard allows students to take quizzes on the go. *Nurse Educator, 28,* 207–209.

Parker, E. B., Riza, L., Tierney, S., & Barrett, A. (2005). Interdisciplinary collaboration: An effective approach for developing Web-based courses. *CIN: Computers, Informatics, Nursing, 23*(6), 308–315.

Patton, C. M., Fedorka, P., & Pavlovich, N. (2004). PhD programs online. In J. J. Fitzpatrick and K. S. Montgomery (Eds.), *Internet for nursing research: A guide to strategies, skills, and resources* (pp. 171–176). New York: Springer Publishing.

Phillips, J. M. (2005). Strategies for active learning in online continuing education. *Journal of Continuing Education in Nursing, 36*(2), 77–83.

Stair, N., & Waltz, C. F. (2004). Web-based graduate research courses. In J. J. Fitzpatrick and K. S. Montgomery (Eds.), *Internet for nursing research: A guide to strategies, skills, and resources* (pp. 157–170). New York: Springer Publishing.

Stella, A., & Gnanam, A. (2004). Quality assurance in distance education: The challenges to be addressed. *Higher Education, 47*(2), 143–160.

Stiles, A. S. (2006). Cooperative learning: Enhancing individual learning through positive group process. In M. H. Oermann & K. Heinrich (Eds.), *Annual review of nursing education* (Vol. 4, pp. 131–159). New York: Springer Publishing.

Chapter 13

ePortfolios in Nursing Education: Not Your Mother's Resume

Janice M. Jones, Kay Sackett, W. Scott Erdley, and John B. Blyth

R esumes have traditionally been used to provide information regarding relevant work experience, educational preparation, awards and honors. For the nursing students at the University at Buffalo (UB), a list of mastered skills is also important when applying for graduate nurse positions, summer internships, and other health care positions. As faculty members, we were frequently called on to write references for students attesting to their clinical skills and academic abilities. However, it soon became apparent that references and resumes displayed only a portion of what nursing students had achieved. This presented increasing challenges after our school of nursing underwent a curriculum change, de-emphasizing experiences in traditional medical-surgical in-hospital care.

To better represent students' skills and talents, our students were first required to develop paper portfolios. After the first semester of implementing this project, we discovered that the paper portfolios were cumbersome for prospective employers to review, difficult for students to mail ahead or carry to interviews, and labor-intensive for faculty to review. When the opportunity presented itself, we shifted students to developing electronic portfolios (or ePortfolios). By preparing an ePortfolio students can communicate their accomplishments and competencies, have an opportunity to work with technology, and demonstrate

This chapter was accepted on April 15, 2006.

their ability to use information technology as a tool. After reviewing the literature, this chapter describes a project that prepared UB nursing students for professional practice in an ever-increasing technologically challenging and complex environment by using a technology-based format showcasing their talents and skills in the form of ePortfolios. In addition, the advantages and disadvantages of implementing ePortfolios are discussed.

What Is an Electronic Portfolio?

A portfolio is "a purposeful collection of assorted work that represents a student's efforts, progress and overall achievements in a course of study" (Karlowicz, 2000, p. 82). Portfolios include work completed over a course of time and are usually organized in chronological order. Portfolios have long been used in the arts and fashion design arena, and only recently in the educational preparation of nurses and teachers (Oermann, 2002; Ryan & Carlton, 1997; Scholes, Webb, Gray, Endacott, Miller, Jasper et al., 2004; Williams, 2001). Although portfolios of the past were in paper or multimedia formats, nursing faculty only recently began using computer-based technologies in the collection, storage, and communication of ePortfolio content.

The ePortfolio has been defined as an "organized collection of digital and/or analog artifacts and reflective statements that demonstrate growth over time" (Treuer & Jensen, 2003, p. 34). ePortfolios are "web-accessible repositories for student work, both graded and ungraded, which may be shared with authorized parties" (Harris & Zastrocky, 2005, p. 8). They use Internet technology, computer technology, networks, and multimedia applications to allow a larger audience access to such a collection of works. In addition, digital technologies can more effectively store, display, and transport portfolio information than their paper counterparts (Ahn, 2004).

History of the ePortfolio in Nursing Education

The application of the ePortfolio to the field of nursing is a relatively recent trend. In the late 1990s, both the National League of Nursing and the American Association of Colleges of Nursing discussed the incorporation of portfolios into nursing education (Ramey & Hay, 2003; Williams, 2001). The American Nurses Association Scope and Standards of Nursing Informatics Practice (2001) complements the National League of Nursing's and the American Association of Colleges of Nursing's perspectives by "supporting the use of information structures, information processes, and information technology" (p. vii) in practice, education, and research. The use of ePortfolios not only provides nursing students an opportunity to collect, organize, and reflect on their work, but also offers an opportunity for nursing educators to evaluate student and program performance. Ramey and Hay (2003) strongly encouraged nursing educators to integrate ePortfolios into baccalaureate curricula to "increase visibility of students' work and accomplishments to audiences within and outside of the nursing profession" (p. 35).

Samples of ePortfolio use in nursing education can be located by conducting a Google™ search using the terms "portfolio" and "ePortfolio." One such search located "Professional Portfolios: Spreadsheet Application" as a portion of a Nursing Informatics course at Kwantlen University College Collaborative Nursing program in British Columbia created by Kaminski (2002). Another search located several examples of a free "Developing a Professional E-Portfolio Workshop Series" for interested students and faculty. These examples suggest ways that technology can assist in evaluating nursing student performance and nursing education programs while positively contributing to the public image of nurses as creative and innovative professionals.

Benefits of ePortfolio Use in Nursing Education

There are many benefits of using ePortfolios in nursing education (Karlowicz, 2000; Ramey & Hay, 2003; Ryan & Carlton, 1997; Williams, 2001). The ability of students to store and share information with anyone regardless of time, place, and over space creates what Treuer and Jenson (2003) term a "virtual identity." Ball, Weaver, and Abbott (2003) suggested that "enabling technologies promise(s) to revitalize the role of nursing in an era of patient safety" (p. 29). ePortfolio documentation of student knowledge and skill acquisition demonstrates preprofessional and professional career development and suggests the adoption of lifelong learning as vital to the enhancement of professional nursing practice.

ePortfolios are valuable for nursing students, nurse educators, program evaluators, and prospective employers. ePortfolios offer nursing students an opportunity to develop critical thinking skills by reflecting on assignments, personal strengths, and weaknesses (Karlowicz, 2000). Developing an ePortfolio allows students the opportunity to document and demonstrate personal and professional growth. Participation in ePortfolio development also encourages students to take greater responsibility for their own learning (Ramey & Hay, 2003) and allows for assessment and reflective practice for students (Bell, 2001; Lettus, Moessner, & Dooley, 2001; Scholes et al., 2004). Students become aware of nursing program goals and how they articulate with individual nursing courses. Lastly, the ePortfolio offers students an opportunity to begin preparing information to include on their resumes and help guide career planning (Williams, 2001). Students are able to reflect on specific clinical and educational experiences to identify areas of interest and future study.

Educators also benefit from the process of student ePortfolio construction. Nursing education faculty may use the ePortfolio as a method of communication with students, as well as a means of fostering student-faculty collaboration. Through reading personal reflections on students' educational experiences, educators are able to evaluate the effectiveness of educational experiences and teaching/learning methodologies, assess student performance and individual learning needs, and make curricular and experiential changes as necessary (Ryan & Carlton, 1997).

Schools of nursing can use student ePortfolios as a method of summative evaluation or program exit assessment to measure a program's effectiveness toward attaining educational and professional objectives (Karlowicz, 2000; Scholes et al., 2004). This type of assessment allows faculty and administrators to connect the competencies of individual nursing courses with the outcomes of the nursing program. In the clinical practice setting, the portfolio can be used as a method of performance appraisal to coincide with a nurse's annual performance review (Thomas, 2005).

Limitations of the ePortfolio in Nursing Education

Although the foregoing highlights the numerous benefits of using student ePortfolios in nursing education, there are limitations of validity, reliability, time, and issues relating to ePortfolio data storage. The use of the student ePortfolio as a means of evaluation in nursing education is limited by a lack of evidence-based research supporting this method as a "valid" method of program and/or student performance. According to Karlowicz (2000), "...no studies indicate that a score assigned to a student portfolio is measuring what it is intended to measure—the acquisition of knowledge and skills necessary for the delivery of competent nursing care" (p. 83). After completion of a 2-year study of portfolio use in nursing education, Scholes and colleagues (2004) recommended that:

- the ePortfolio needs to link theory and practice
- there needs to be a clear fit between the ePortfolio and professional practice to be evaluated
- the outcomes evaluated should be consistent with the students' professional and academic development (p. 596).

A second limitation of the use of student ePortfolios as a method of evaluation is the lack of interrater reliability. The fair and equal rating of student ePortfolios is limited by a lack of standardization in the organization and substance of the portfolios. Although the content of the student's ePortfolio may be similar, the variations in design and presentation make assigning a grade to such a project difficult.

Time is another limitation in the use of ePortfolios. The construction and evaluation of nursing student ePortfolios require a substantial amount of time for students, faculty, technology support staff, and administration. In addition to the time needed to develop and create templates or purchase and evaluate software applications, implement the project, develop standards, evaluate the process, and secure server space for warehousing the ePortfolio, the use of ePortfolios requires the acknowledgment of a learning curve. Time must be devoted to students, faculty, staff, and administration familiarizing themselves with the use of software applications and web-based technology.

Lastly, storage and maintenance of ePortfolio information presents a limitation to the widespread use of the ePortfolio in nursing education. This is a vital concern when considering the use of ePortfolios as the digital storage of information over time presents unique financial, legal, and security issues for institutions of higher education. Students may house their ePortfolios utilizing the university's Web space, but problems arise once the student graduates and no longer has this "free space" available.

The Beginnings: The Technology and the Process

In the spring of 2003, the director of Science and Engineering Node Services (SENS) at UB, the assistant director of academic services/chief information officer, and an instructional support specialist for SENS were awarded a Faculty Educational Technology Grant from the university for development of an ePortfolio system. This ePortfolio would allow students to collect artifacts representing their academic work and collegiate experiences at UB. An introduction to ePortfolio use at the UB School of Nursing is found at http://nursing.buffalo.edu/eportfolio/index.asp.

In a large, comprehensive, research institution, where lower division students take many large-enrollment classes, it is important to ensure that students see "the big picture" of their educational experience. The goal of this project was to help undergraduate students reflect on their undergraduate career, course work, learning experiences, progress toward a degree, intellectual growth, and future career goals. The original purpose of this project was to develop a way for students to preserve examples of their work and distribute it to others, especially prospective employers.

The objectives of this collaborative project included the following:

- deliver a stand-alone cross-platform application (works well on Windows, Macintosh, UNIX, and Linux operating systems)
- design a web-based cross-browser compatible application compliant with the recommendations of the World Wide Web Consortium (W3C), and
- develop a project that was complete and ready for students to use by the beginning of the 2004 fall semester.

The complete report on the development of the project can be found at http://www.eng.buffalo.edu/Projects/eportfolio/report/.

The initial ePortfolio CD, primarily developed by graduate students employed in the university's Electronic Technology Center (ETC), was released by ETC and called "UB ePortfolio Alpha Version 1.1." The technology platform chosen for this model was Macromedia Flash. For the program to function as a template for students, the graduate students manually completed much of the programming code. This method ultimately proved to be inefficient when the ePortfolio was first released.

Much of the intended functionality of the program was inoperable, including the ability to add links in the ePortfolio. The CD released by ETC had a self-installing function that enabled students to "easily" begin designing their ePortfolio within minutes of starting the program. One of the main features of the program, the ability to self-publish the completed work, did not function at the time of release. An Alpha Version 1.2 was developed in the hopes of fixing these problems.

In the summer of 2004, the authors and the SENS persons discussed the possibility of pilot testing Version 1.2 of the original template. It was determined that a small group of students would be ideal for initial testing of the application, even though the application was not without its problems. The group selected was an initial cohort of nursing students, approximately 17 in number, in a new accelerated baccalaureate nursing program. The original timeline called for the pilot test with this cohort to take place in the first session of the summer of 2004 with analysis and revision during the second session (Figure 13.1). The revised version was to be rolled out with the incoming traditional junior nursing students

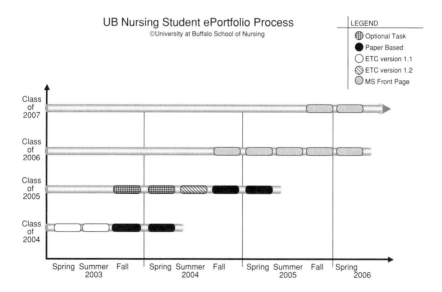

FIGURE 13.1   Timeline of ePortfolio construction.
Source: Reprinted by permission of the University at Buffalo School of Nursing, April 12, 2006.

in the 2004 fall semester, with analysis and revisions during subsequent semesters as necessary. This timetable would allow for a phasing-in type of adoption. The initial group of senior nursing students would continue with pen and paper portfolio format through their graduation.

All parties briefly considered the potential of using the university's course management system (Blackboard®). However, after assessing this possibility, the system was determined to not have the necessary features, at that time, for the application. Therefore, the plan for a stand-alone application moved forward. The decision to explore other options for the nursing students resulted in several weeks of testing open-source programs and researching what other universities were using.

Implementation Problems

The implementation did not proceed as smoothly as anticipated, and a number of impediments emerged. The first was the application distribution that was behind schedule and was related to a problem burning the application to the CDs. This required a few weeks to successfully resolve. The second issue was poor compatibility of the application with student and faculty computers. Many students were unable to perform clean installs on their personal computers, whereas the installation would only work on MS-Windows machines. There was incompatibility related to the different Windows operating system versions on student computers. One of the faculty had her laptop completely crash as a result of the installation. There were user issues that extended beyond the installation process. Even though the accelerated baccalaureate students in the original pilot cohort were fairly well-versed in using computers, they quickly became quite frustrated with the application because of the installation issues and inability to work on their respective ePortfolio at different locations.

In spite of these difficulties, it was determined that implementation would move forward with the traditional junior students in the 2004 fall semester. The problems outlined previously, even though addressed to some degree by the developers, multiplied greatly because of the increased number of students using the application. After working with the application, students strongly resisted change. One faculty member and the technical support person ended up dealing with most of the students on these issues. The time devoted to providing support and instruction far outweighed the advantages of the application. Faculty and our web specialist continue to provide support for students along with assistance from peers who feel more comfortable with the program and process related to the ePortfolio.

The FrontPage™ ePortfolio Template Is Born

Diez (1996) viewed the ePortolio as a map; a portfolio provides a framework for one to look at where next to set goals for one's own progress (p. 23). Diez's map metaphor reflected the basis for choosing an application, namely one that can be easily changed by the student to reflect their evolving educational process. Given the many imperfections and problems associated with the initial release of the software, an alternate method of developing a template was explored by the School of Nursing (SON) faculty associated with this project. It was at this stage that Microsoft FrontPage was chosen as the program for creating the SON ePortfolio template. A major factor affecting this decision was the UB Microsoft Campus Agreement, which allows students to purchase a personal copy of the FrontPage program for a simple user fee of $4.95 at the university computer store.

The original stand-alone application was a tabular organized screen with the tabs listed in horizontal fashion across the top of the screen. Each user could change the descriptor used for each tab. The new FrontPage template consists of five basic pages in a navigational layout that is easily interpreted by the designing student and the prospective employer visiting a student's online ePortfolio. These sections encompass the:

1. *Introduction*: an area of the ePortfolio that introduces the student by means of a brief biography in essay form (Figure 13.2)
2. *Resume*: a section for uploading students' current version of this document
3. *Nursing Skills Proficiency Tests*: a section listing nursing students' skills acquired thus far (Figure 13.3)
4. *Academic achievements*: an area to showcase presentations and academic works (Figure 13.4)
5. *Contact form*: an area that allows the web visitor to contact the student via form to e-mail.

What do you want to be when you grow up?

I've always had difficulty answering the question, "What do you want to be when you grow up?" Since I was young, I've gone through a wide array of professions including, an astronaut, a clown and a teacher. Looking back those ideas may have seemed outrageous, but there was a reason for each career choice. I wanted to be an astronaut to explore the world, I wanted to be a clown to make people laugh and smile, and I wanted to be a teacher to help others learn. Although I chose a much different path than I had expected, I am thrilled to be where I am today. In May of 2003, I graduated with a BS in psychology from Baldwin-Wallace College in Berea, OH. After graduation it was then that I decided to follow my heart into a career that had always been of interest to me. I've always looked up to my mother who has been a nurse for over 30 years.

FIGURE 13.2   Introduction with brief biography of student.

Source: Reprinted by permission of the University at Buffalo School of Nursing, April 12, 2006.

NURSING SKILLS

I have mastered many of the skills required for the nursing profession and my mastery level has been demonstrated through many skills proficiency tests.

For example: I have mastered the administration of medication whether oral or via injections (IM and SQ).
Calculations were demonstrated to administer the proper dose to the client, both adult and pediatric.
The medications were given following the six rights (right client, right route, right time, and documentation).
The medications involved inhalers, ointments, eye drops, ear drops, skin patches, cream, powder, enemas, etc.

Other skills that I have mastered and demonstrated include:

Vital signs- Which include blood pressure, pulse, temperatur and respiratory monitoring.
Use Nurse Process- Assessing the patient, identify a problem, planning, intervention and evaluations.
Veni-puncture- Discontinuing IV's
Catheterization- Both internal and external catheter
Surgical Dressing- Either with Staples or steri-strips
Surgical Asepsis- Maintaining sterility to decrease infection
Trach. Care- Using sterile technique
Suctioning- To help patient with a trach. who is unable to expectorate, cyanotic, precedence of crackles or wheezes
Finger stick- To monitor the patient's blood glucose level (Diabetes Mellitus)
Mobility / ROM Exercises- For all patients (especially those who are at bed rest)

FIGURE 13.3   Skills proficiency tests or listing of skills.

Source: Reprinted by permission of the University at Buffalo School of Nursing, April 12, 2006.

Achievements:

I am a member of the nursing honor society, Sigma Theta Tau International, Gamma Kappa Chapter.
I was presented with two Staff Commendation Reports while working as a Unit Clerk at Heathwood. One for "Exceptional kindness to resident or family member" and one for "Exceptional work performance in difficult situation."

Examples of my Academic Work:

Philosophy of Nursing - Spring 2006
Evidence Based Project - Spring 2006
This research project was done using current research to support our theory that laboring mothers have better outcomes with good labor support.
Organizational Analysis - Fall 2005
This paper was done to evaluate the organizational structure of a medical/surgical floor.
Comprehensive Assessment - Spring 2005
This paper was done as part of my primary care clinical experience. It includes a health history, complete physical, and nutritional and health risk assessments.
Community Assessment - Spring 2005
This paper is a community assessment of the Village of Williamsville, a small portion of Amherst, NY.
Fiscal Project PowerPoint Presentation - Spring 2005
I created this presentation to supplement a proposal for the Western New York VNA to revamp their cell phone reimbursement policy.
Health History - Fall 2004
I interviewed the subject of this paper and used that information to prepare this health history. The components include her chief complaint, HPI, past medical history, family history, and review of systems. It also includes a genogram.
Health Risk Appraisal - Fall 2004
I performed a Health Risk Appraisal online with the subject of the paper. It identified several areas where he could change health behaviors to improve his overall health status. Interventions were developed and a plan was put into place to improve one behavior, increasing fiber intake, and a contract was signed to help keep the subject on track.

FIGURE 13.4   Academic achievements.

Source: Reprinted by permission of the University at Buffalo School of Nursing, April 12, 2006.

The generic template was uploaded to the SON Web site along with a set of step-by-step instructions. Similarly, a frequently asked questions section was also created and uploaded for student access. These tools, along with a 2-hour orientation in the school's computer laboratory, comprised the basis for the nursing student to begin designing their ePortfolio. The majority of nursing students found the creation of the FrontPage ePortfolio to be relatively painless. The ability to work with the Microsoft FrontPage software became second nature to students experienced with Microsoft Word™. Technical support was available to students experiencing difficulty with the program and usually on an as-needed, one-to-one basis. Additional support was provided to students by utilizing the university online course management system powered by Blackboard and designated UBlearns (http://ublearns.buffalo.edu). Each class cohort was enrolled in a support course where blog-type discussion boards were used to assist students having technical problems with the software. One such problem was how to publish students' final work to their personal Web space provided by the university.

Where We Are Now

The majority of the implementation problems encountered were associated with the initial ETC developed application and decreased greatly once the FrontPage template came into use. Students start the ePortfolio in their first semester of the nursing program and add to their ePortfolio each subsequent semester. The first semester forms the basis for the ePortfolio. The ePortfolio at this level consists of an introduction, a resume, a list of nursing skills, honors and awards, certificates earned such as HIPAA (the Health Insurance Portability and Accountability Act) and CPR, and one or two examples of a paper or PowerPoint presentation. In the second and third semesters, the resume is updated; the students' nursing philosophy is added; the list of skills is updated along with any honors, awards, and certificates earned. Students are encouraged to include PowerPoint presentations along with a fiscal analysis and organizational culture/job satisfaction analysis. The management course in the last semester of the program prepares students for their first professional nursing position. Mock interviews are conducted with the Career Planning and Placement Office, and the ePortfolio is refined to represent graduate nurses seeking employment in a variety of settings. The ePortfolio is uploaded to the student's Web site for easy access by a prospective employer. The traditional resume may also be uploaded to an employment site with a link to the student's Web site embedded in the resume.

The final endpoint repository for the project is projected to be the University's Career Planning and Placement Department hosting the completed ePortfolios for students after graduation. This will allow for employer access and student use during the employment process.

Evaluation and Expansion of the Project

The goal of this project is to propel nursing students into the 21st century using a technology-based format showcasing their talents and skills. The ePortfolio operationalizes this goal, and the evaluation process is ongoing as students continue to use and develop their ePortfolios. As the ePortfolio is used throughout each semester, students continue to need "refresher classes" in downloading and uploading their ePortfolios as they update them via course assignments. The difficulties encountered with students learning the application are now minimal and usually result from the student's lack of preparation in developing the ePortfolio (e.g., following basic directions and instructions). Having an "ePortfolio course" on Blackboard has diminished many problematic areas. We continue to respond to student questions through e-mail, discussions on Blackboard, and individual or group sessions when needed. Although initial orientation to the ePortfolio requires some time in explaining the project and the software, students come to require less guidance as they continue to work through the template each semester.

Initially introduced to undergraduate students, we are attempting to incorporate ePortfolios into the master's and doctoral programs. The ePortfolio may be converted into a curriculum vitae for those needing such documentation. Of special note, responses from employers have been mixed, with some human resource personnel in awe of the student's presentation of skills, whereas others continue to request only the traditional paper-based resume.

Conclusion

The project described in this chapter focuses on preparing students for professional practice in an ever-increasing technologically challenging and complex environment. Preparing an ePortfolio not only provides students an opportunity to work with technology, but it also demonstrates, to prospective employers, an ability to utilize information technology as a tool. As this chapter illustrates, ePortfolios are the wave of the future, and innovative nurse educators would do well to consider extending this opportunity to their undergraduate and graduate students. Faculty need to be aware though of the potential pitfalls and impediments related to implementation.

REFERENCES

Ahn, J. (2004). Electronic portfolios: Blending technology, accountability & assessment. *T.H.E. Journal, 4*, 12–18.

American Nurses Association. (2001). *Scope and standards of nursing informatics practice.* Washington, DC: ANA.

Ball, M. J., Weaver, C., & Abbott, P. A. (2003). Enabling technologies promise to revitalize the role of nursing in an era of patient safety. *The Journal of Medical Informatics, 69,* 29–38.

Bell, S. (2001). Professional nurse's portfolio. *Nursing Administration Quarterly, 25*(2), 69–73.

Diez, M. (1996). The portfolio: Sonnet, mirror and map. In K. Burke (Ed.), *Professional portfolios* (p. 23). Arlington Heights, VA: IRI Skylight.

Harris, M., & Zastrocky, M. (2005). *Gartner industry research hype cycle for higher education, 2005.* ID Number G00130295, 1–13.

Kaminski, J. (2002). *Kwantlen University College Bachelor's of Science in Nursing Program: Nursing informatics: Professional portfolios: Spreadsheet application.* Retrieved May 28, 2003, from http://www.nursing-informatics.com/kwantlen/nrsg1241.html

Karlowicz, K. A. (2000). The value of student portfolios to evaluate undergraduate nursing programs. *Nurse Educator, 25*(2), 73–78.

Lettus, M. K., Moessner, P. M., & Dooley, L. (2001). The clinical portfolio as an assessment tool. *Nursing Administration Quarterly, 25*(2), 74–79.

Oermann, M. H. (2002). Developing a professional portfolio in Nursing. *Orthopedic Nursing, 21*(2), 73–78.

Ramey, S. L, & Hay, M. L. (2003). Using electronic portfolios to measure student achievement and assess curricular integrity. *Nurse Educator, 28*(1), 31–36.

Ryan, M., & Carlton, K. H. (1997). Portfolio applications in a school of nursing. *Nurse Educator, 22*(1), 35–39.

Scholes, J., Webb, C., Gray, M., Endacott, R., Miller, C., Jaspar, M., & McMullan, M. (2004). Uses and innovations in nursing education: Making portfolios work in practice. *Journal of Advanced Nursing, 46,* 595–603.

Thomas, D. O. (2005). A better response to performance reviews. *RN, 68*(4), 44–46.

Treuer, P., & Jenson, J. D. (2003). Electronic portfolios need standards to thrive. *Educause Quarterly, 2,* 34–42.

Williams, J. (2001). The clinical notebook: Using student portfolios to enhance clinical teaching and learning. *Journal of Nursing Education, 40,* 135–137.

Chapter 14

"How Can I Fail the NCLEX-RN® With a 3.5 GPA?": Approaches to Help This Unexpected High-Risk Group

Paulette Demaske Rollant

Ask nursing educators: "Who are the high-risk students?" They will tell you, "Those students who have less than a 3.0 GPA." It is true that many of the students I tutored over the past 23 years were those with less than 3.0 GPAs who needed to "get up to speed" to pass school tests or the NCLEX-RN® examinations. However, many students I tutored who failed the NCLEX-RN, not only on the initial but on numerous attempts, were students with high GPAs throughout their program. Over the past 3 to 4 years, this unique group has grown.

Background

The academic and nonacademic factors that influence nursing students' success on the licensure examination have been widely reported. The majority of studies focus on the predictors for success and not specific interventions (Beeson & Kissling, 2001; Foti & DeYoung, 1992; McClelland, Yang, & Glick, 1992; Seldomridge & DiBartolo, 2004; Waterhouse, Bucher, & Beeman, 1994; Yin & Burger, 2003). Most of these studies focus on objective data, such as preadmissions standards,

This chapter was accepted on April 10, 2006.

progression examinations, overall grade point average, course grades, and comprehensive examinations. Crow, Handley, Morrison, and Shelton (2004) concluded after conducting a national survey of 513 generic BSN programs that the use of standardized entrance and content mastery examinations support the ability to assess readiness for the NCLEX-RN.

Seven significant predictor variables for passing the NCLEX-RN were identified by Beeman and Waterhouse (2001). The total number of C+ or lower grades earned in nursing theory courses was the best predictor, followed by grades in several individual nursing courses. Ninety-four percent of "passes" were correctly classified, as were 92% of NCLEX-RN failures. The authors stated that this degree of accuracy for failures represented improvement over results reported in previous studies.

However, many questions remain as to why certain candidates fail the examination, especially when they have indicators that predict their success to pass. Beeman and Waterhouse (2003) conducted a pilot study to explore postgraduation influences on the NCLEX-RN. They used a newly developed NCLEX Preparation Survey that explored factors such as length and type of study, work hours, review course participation, sleep, and stress. Results suggested both expected and unexpected relationships between these factors and NCLEX-RN mastery.

Other studies have also examined factors that influence achievement on the NCLEX-RN. Arathuzik and Aber (1998) published results of a study, using a descriptive correlational design, with senior nursing students enrolled in a generic program in an urban public university. The results highlighted several internal and external blocks to success as described by the students (e.g., family responsibilities, emotional distress, fatigue, and financial/work burdens). Significant correlations were found between success on the NCLEX-RN and five factors: cumulative nursing program grade point average, English as the primary language spoken at home, lack of family responsibilities or demands, lack of emotional distress, and sense of competency in critical thinking. They recommended the establishment of a comprehensive database, including factors associated with success in the NCLEX-RN and programs of advisement, tutoring, and stress management, as well as classes in study skills, test taking, and NCLEX-RN preparation.

Wood (2005) concluded that to be successful on the NCLEX-RN students need both knowledge of the nursing content as well as familiarity and comfort with the technology used during the examination.

DiBartolo and Seldomridge (2005) reported their findings from an integrative literature review of intervention studies used in baccalaureate programs to improve NCLEX-RN passes. Researchers identified being limited in their ability to attribute success specifically to the interventions. They recommended further investigation using more rigorous designs with larger, diverse student groups to evaluate both type and timing of various interventions. Frith, Sewell, and Clark (2005) described how best practices associated with a change to computerized testing and more in-depth test preparation enhanced students' opportunities for success and reduced stress among faculty.

In summary, the literature provides information on predictors and tools to identify students who are at risk for failure on the NCLEX-RN. It also indicates the importance of other factors—such as fatigue and anxiety—on passing the NCLEX-RN. This chapter presents interventions used by the author for the past 23 years to prepare students for the licensure examination and for taking other tests in nursing programs. Successful test-takers, as well as graduates of nursing schools during tutoring, have offered support of the actions and approaches described in this chapter.

"How Can I Fail the NCLEX-RN With a 3.5 GPA?"

Why is it that students with high GPAs are failing their NCLEX-RN? My hunch is that these students with high GPAs do well enough in school to restate the information back on tests. They are test wise, that is, they get to know "how a teacher tests." Although, in most instances, they "know" the answers on the test items, they have little experience in the critical thinking skills area of: how do I "figure it out when I don't know?". Therefore, they lack the processing tools to make an educated guess or to look at factors beyond content knowledge. What these students with high GPAs do lack is an approach to test-taking that I describe as, "I will go with what I know" (Rollant, 1988, 2006).

Having worked with these unique, high-risk students during their academic programs, they show little interest in learning new ways to approach testing because they do not think they need them. In the same vein, some educators regard this "figure it out" approach to answering test questions as controversial. They argue that the students just need to know the content. The counter argument is, of course, that in clinical practice nurses do not and will not know all the content and will have to figure some things out. This chapter describes two self-report inventories I have found useful for tracking and predicting risk for failure or success on tests and the NCLEX-RN: the Test Anxiety Inventory (TAI) and the Learning Assessment Study Skills Inventory (LASSI), along with two critical subjective questions and questions adapted from my "5 C's for Success Model." In addition, actions to initiate within the first 2 to 3 months of a nursing program and implications for nurse educators are shared.

Test Anxiety Inventory: What It Is and How to Use It

The TAI, a self-report scale, measures individual differences in test anxiety as a situation-specific trait. Grounded in state-trait anxiety theory, this one-page test contains 20 items that asks respondents to indicate how frequently they experience specific symptoms of anxiety before, during, and after examinations. The subscales also assess worry and emotionality as major components of test anxiety (Spielberger et al., 1990).

Rather than using the TAI to measure different types of anxiety levels, I use the scores to determine the number of mental and physical activities the test-takers need to practice and use during examinations. For example, depending on a student's score, I might recommend two mental activities:

- Recite the affirmation, "I know something," three times every 2 hours throughout the day.
- Close eyes before getting out of bed and picture a pleasant scene from the prior week for at least 1 minute.

For physical activities, I might recommend the practice of taking three slow and deep breaths:

- Inhale via the nose for a count of four.
- Hold for a count of two.
- Exhale fully via the mouth to a count of four.
- Place a hand on abdomen to see the hand rise and fall for correct abdominal breathing.

For a second physical exercise, I often suggest the following sequence as a way of helping students relax prior to and during a test:

- Curl the toes tightly as if holding onto the floor.
- Tighten muscle groups in an ascending manner until the entire body is tense.
- Hold muscle groups of the entire body tense for 3 to 5 seconds.
- Release all muscle groups into relaxation.

Students with the most difficulties are often those who do not see a need for learning these strategies or are so tense that they have poor physical and mental control.

When I administer the TAI, I add a question about anxiety around taking tests on a computer. Those who indicate a high score on this item are at risk to fail simply because of their anxiety with computer testing. Often, they fear they will run out of time. I give these students five questions with a timer set for 5 minutes. After a few days, the number of questions is increased by five questions and so on. In this way, their confidence in having enough time to answer questions increases.

Learning Assessment Study Skills Inventory: What It Is and How to Use It

The Learning Assessment Study Skills Inventory (LASSI) is an 80-item assessment of students' awareness about and their use of learning and study strategies. The results are related to the skill, will, and self-regulation components of strategic learning. This valid and reliable assessment inventory contains 10 scales: stress, attitude, motivation, concentration, self testing, time management, test-taking skills, anxiety, information processing, and study aids. The focus of the Inventory is on behaviors, attitudes, and beliefs related to successful learning. The LASSI provides students with an assessment of their strengths and weaknesses and feedback about how to improve (Weinstein, Schulte, & Palmer, 1990).

Initially, I use the results of the LASSI to pinpoint specific areas for remediation. What is interesting is that, if a student makes changes in one or two of the scales, it influences the other scales. I find this helps students not to get overwhelmed with a few new actions.

A second use is to determine the risk of failure based on groupings of extreme high or low percentile scores. Since the mid-1990's, I have used the LASSI to track NCLEX-RN test-takers for success. Initially, I identified that graduates with four or more of the 10 scales at or below the 50th percentile were at risk for failure. This group sometimes reported seeing no need to change actions for test preparation or during tests. The group with the 10 scales between the 50th and the 70th percentiles seemed to be more receptive to suggested changes and more often implemented specific actions with results of test success. Some of the students reported that the addition of one or two new actions based on a LASSI scale that had a lower percentile score resulted in success on the NCLEX-RN.

In a retrospective study, I discovered test-takers with four or more scales over the 70th percentile had failed the NCLEX-RN. This group more commonly had 4.0 GPAs. My hunch was that they were over-confident, because they did well in school and knew the content. They saw no need to do anything different and were strongly resistant to making test behavior changes. Thus, when they found something they did not know during the test, their first action was panic, which later turned into apathy. Several graduates who fell into this category and failed the NCLEX-RN shared with me that they "just wanted to get out of there." When I worked with them for specific test-taking skills after their NCLEX-RN failure, they made a few changes in reading processes and passed. Afterward, a number admitted, "I wish I would have done this before. I could have used these actions."

Critical Subjective Questions

Another approach for assessing students for high risk is to ask seniors to write their responses to two questions near the end of their last semester:

- Explain how doing two daily mental and physical actions the week before the NCLEX-RN will enhance your preparation for the test.
- Discuss one mental and one physical action you will use *during* the NCLEX-RN.

In one school, about 5 years ago, I reviewed how seniors at the end of the last semester answered these questions. Interestingly, the only two failures on the NCLEX-RN were students with high GPAs who answered these questions with "you need to..." instead of "I need to...."

Since that time, I have found that this exercise of critical subjective questions acts as an informal assessment for the risk of failure on the NCLEX-RN. I believe it raises a "yellow flag" that students believe they know the content and do not need to prepare for the examination, especially with mental or physical relaxation exercises.

Questions Based on the "5 C's for Test Success"

A final self-report assessment for risk of failure on the NCLEX-RN is the use of questions based on my model, The "5 C's for Test Success" (Rollant, 1988, 2006). In 1988, I developed an initial model of "4 C's for Test Success" on the NCLEX-RN, with equal emphasis given to each piece of the model—content, control, confidence, common sense. Since that time, I prioritized the components—content, confidence, control, and common sense—and added a fifth component "compare." Also, I established that all of them are interconnected and provide alerts for graduates to use in preparation for and during the NCLEX-RN. The model allows for individual and group analysis for test preparation and specific actions based on the respondents' perceptions. "The 5 C's for Test Success" (Rollant, 2006) include:

1. Content
2. Confidence, e.g., "I know something. I will figure it out, and I will go with what I KNOW" (Rollant, 1983)
3. Control of (a) Tension—initial and later, (b) Fatigue, and (c) Loss of Focus
4. Common sense
5. Compare, for example, an answer with the reworded question or compare options when narrowed to two options.

Faculty can use this model in preparing students for the NCLEX-RN. For example, educators can ask students at the end of every term the questions listed below. This can be done in a discussion with students or by asking students to write their answers on index cards, with or without their names. These questions encourage students to think about the test beyond the content that will be evaluated.

1. Content—"Do you know the content?"
2. Confidence—"What do you know?" and "What are you going to do?"
3. Control
   a. "Do you get tense at the beginning or end of the test?"
   b. "Do you get an "attitude" when you get tired, such as, "I just want to get out of here! I don't care!'"
   c. "Do you get bored or "lose focus" on the test?"
   d. "At what question number do you get bored?"
4. Common Sense—"What does your common sense tell you the answer might be?"
5. Compare
   a. "Do you confirm your answer to the question before you go to the next question?"
   b. "When you narrow options to two, do you compare them before deciding?" (Rollant, 2006).

The responses to these questions can guide actions to use with students to raise their confidence in taking the NCLEX-RN.

Actions to Use Early On

Reinforce Confidence

Confidence is the critical component in the "5 C's for Test Success" model. Unfortunately, when graduates take nursing tests and the NCLEX-RN, this component is often their least well developed. When I ask students or graduates at NCLEX-RN reviews, "Do you have the content to pass NCLEX-RN?," they respond with a "yes," "maybe," and "no." For this reason, I have them complete a physical action and state "yes" loudly and enthusiastically. Because a part of passing the NCLEX-RN is confidence, I repeat this activity at the beginning, middle, and end of my interactions with them. To reinforce the test-taking skills of "I know something" and "I have tools to figure it out when I don't know," I recommend that educators ask this question before examinations or at the end of each class and challenge students to respond with an enthusiastic "Yes!" (Rollant, 2006).

Counter Boredom or Loss of Focus

Strategies are needed to counter boredom and loss of focus during examinations. In the past year, about 20% of my groups of students preparing for the NCLEX-RN reported to get bored between questions16 to 20. Another 70% get bored between questions 25 to 35, and only about 5 to 10% report the ability to progress to question 50 without boredom.

When I ask educators, "At what question do your students get bored during a test?," their response is a look of surprise. They sometimes respond: "My students don't have that problem." I challenge educators to ask students that question during test reviews. Then, before each test, remind students to identify when they get bored and to use an action to deal with it. Some simple actions would be to reposition in their seat, smile, close their eyes, take three slow deep breaths, as well as change their reading process to include test-taking skills (Figure 14.1) and do muscle group exercises.

What are the consequences of boredom? This underlying loss of focus typically explodes into an attitude change of "I don't care," especially on tests longer than 50 items. This attitude change may lead to a change of perception about what the questions ask and how options are read (i.e., misreading the items). I have found that misreading the questions and options is a frequent cause of wrong answers.

Practice by students while in school for "awareness and actions" to fight the loss of focus enhances success on the NCLEX-RN. Graduates feel confident to have tools to use when examinations are more than 75 questions. Educators also might consider giving one long test, e.g., 265 items similar to the maximum number of items on the NCLEX-RN, during which the students are coached every 25 questions about how to minimize loss of focus.

Compare

Compare is the third action strategy. Students are encouraged to compare the selected option with a rephrased question. When students are

Skill 1: Compare...
- Your answer to the "reworded" question
- What you think versus see?
- What is the question asking versus the selected options? Is it asking priority or that three options are incorrect and one correct?

Skill 2: Reword ... the Question
- Use "I"
- Use your own and easy-to-understand words

Skill 3: Define "What is the Problem?"
- Are time frames important?
- What is the body system?
- What is a complication of the problem?
- If it is nurse centered – think nursing process – assessment before interventions
- If it is client need centered – think Maslow – physiologic before psychosocial needs

Skill 4: Compare - Options
- How are they different?
- How are they similar?
- Is a time frame given in each? Is it important?
- Can you use labels or a category for each option, eg, actual/potential or subjective/objective? For all four options or when narrowed to two?

FIGURE 14.1   Test-taking skills.
Source: © 2006 Rollant Concepts, Inc. Reprinted by permission of Paulette D. Rollant, April 5, 2006.

completing practice questions, the educator can suggest that they read the question and options out loud to hear how they would change the question or the options. A critical action during question rephrasing is to use "I should... " instead of "the nurse should.... " Test-takers will often err by mentally changing the question once they get to the last option. Students report that this one action of comparing the selected option to a rephrased question is highly effective in helping them decide on the correct answer to the item.

The second way in which the compare strategy works is for students to change their reading processes (e.g., to review the options to see how they are different and how they are similar then label each with a theme or to rephrase the question). Potential effective themes or labels for options include actual/potential, acute/chronic, or specific/general.

Successful test-takers reported that, when they narrowed the options to two, labeling them and then comparing them individually to the rephrased question was most helpful. For example, if the options are narrowed to two, and the stem asks "which patient should be seen first," by labeling the options as acute or chronic, students are guided to select the acute problem, which is usually tended to first (Figure 14.2).

Show Them What They Do Not Know

Based on posttest interviews, written and oral, I have learned that small, yet specific, actions based on an individual's errors in reading or thinking may make the difference between passing and failing. When individuals use one or two tools that produce positive results, their confidence increases significantly. If individuals are confident, they will approach the test questions with an enthusiastic attitude of "I can figure it out. I know something, and I will go with what I know" (Rollant, 2006).

What Does This Mean for Educators in Nursing?

Know Your Students

These actions will enhance the familiarity of your students:

1. In the initial week of the term, consider giving students a 30-item examination with application and analysis questions. This helps all levels of students recognize their need to prepare for the examination.
2. Initiate test-taking skills the initial week of *each* semester with the use of the 30-item examination.
3. Review the preassessments, often given as preadmission tests, that are currently being implemented at your school for each class (e.g., on learning abilities and styles, skills, and prior experiences in nursing). Ask what stress management actions students use outside of school and build on these for test-taking.
4. Assess students' level of boredom and anxiety with testing. When do they have these feelings—at the beginning, middle, or end of the test? At what number test question?

Practice for options: do 15 minutes daily

- Cover the question
- Read options first and in a sequence of
  - 4 to 1 or
  - 1 to 4
- Compare the options as you read them
- Label them
- Ask if priority is important – if yes, then approach the options as all of them being correct and place them in order of priority
- Ask what if I did – didn't – then what?
- Do not look at the question

Practice for questions: do 15 minutes daily

- Cover the options
- Read the question
- Rephrase the question in "I" format
- Key in on the clues of time, age, location
- Ask what is the "BIG PICTURE"?
- Make a story about the stem
- Use simple words – substitute age groups ages (e.g., toddler for a 4-year-old) or the word "medication" for unknown names of medications
- Ask yourself: What do I know?
- Identify if the question is a priority where the *best* of 4 correct options is to be selected or if one correct answer is the task
- Do not look at the options

FIGURE 14.2 Different ways to read test items

Source: ©2006 Rollant Concepts, Inc. Reprinted by permission of Paulette Demaske Rollant, April 5, 2006.

Map Your Processes

Below are some actions that will enhance your interactions with students in helping them prepare for the NCLEX-RN.

1. Become knowledgeable about the NCLEX-RN test plan.
2. Map your objectives, content, and tests with the test plan.
3. Change your teaching strategies to fit your group. How you taught the last group may be less effective with a future group of students. What portion of your classes are visual, auditory and tactile learners? Adapt your presentation style to each group.
4. Conduct test reviews with focus on test-taking skills.
5. Include physical and mental preparation, as well as review of the content.

Make NCLEX-RN Real

Students should have experience with NCLEX-RN–type questions as they progress through the nursing curriculum. They can take periodic quizzes in the program and monitor their progress with these items. Students should become familiar with the test plan and can be directed to http://www.ncsbn.org early in a nursing program. Students can be assigned the task of rewriting a question and comparing a set of options. This activity might be done at the beginning of each class a number of times in a course or as an online activity. The educator should relate these practice questions with the content examined in that unit or that day. Sample test items should be reviewed and discussed with students in terms of test-taking skills.

Test-Taking Tips to Review With Students

Some additional test-taking strategies to review with students are:

1. Include 1 to 2 minutes of "focus" time before *each* test. Ask students to close their eyes and either think of nothing or mentally picture something pleasant.

2. Remind them to ask themselves, "What do I know?" throughout tests rather than, "I don't know this. I never heard of this."
3. Give students a blank index card to write on during the test. They can draw something positive for confidence or record content they fear they will forget during the test. Collect the index cards after the test. In addition to benefiting students, this is a great way to evaluate content or issues that are of concern or confusing to them.

Summary

Individuals who fail the NCLEX-RN include students with low and high GPAs. Over the past several years, I have found that the group with the high GPAs has increased in numbers. This chapter described selected assessment tools, as well as unique questions, to help educators and students track and assess "risk" for failure on tests—the NCLEX-RN in particular. Actions for educators to take with students include the following:

- reinforcing confidence,
- countering loss of focus/boredom, and
- teaching the comparison method.

All of these methods are taken from the "5 Cs for Test Success" model (Rollant, 2006). The final action is to help students identify tools to use when they do not know. Using these strategies, educators can open the pathway to success for students at potential risk for test failure.

REFERENCES

Arathuzik, D., & Aber, C. (1998). Factors associated with national council licensure examination-registered nurse success. *Journal of Professional Nursing, 14*(2), 119–126.

Beeman, P., & Waterhouse, J. (2001). NCLEX-RN performance: Predicting success on the computerized examination. *Journal of Professional Nursing, 17*, 158–165.

Beeman, P., & Waterhouse, J. (2003). Post-graduation factors predicting NCLEX-RN® success. *Nurse Educator, 28*(6), 257–260.

Beeson, S., & Kissling, G. (2001). Predicting success for baccalaureate graduates on the NCLEX-RN. *Journal of Professional Nursing, 17*(3), 121–127.

Crow, C., Handley, M., Morrison, R., & Shelton, M. (2004). Requirements and interventions used by BSN programs to promote and predict NCLEX-RN success: A national study. *Journal of Professional Nursing, 20*(3), 174–186.

DiBartolo, M. C, & Seldomridge, L. A. (2005). Review of intervention studies to promote NCLEX-RN success of baccalaureate students. *Nurse Educator, 30*(4), 166–171.

Foti, I., & DeYoung, S. (1992). Predicting success on the National Council Licensure Examination–Registered Nurse: Another piece of the puzzle. *Journal of Professional Nursing, 7*(2), 99–104.

Frith, K., Sewell, J., & Clark, D. (2005). Best practices in NCLEX-RN readiness preparation for baccalaureate student success. *CIN: Computers, Informatics, Nursing, 23*(6), 322–329.

McClelland, E., Yang, J., & Glick, O. (1992). A statewide study of academic variables affecting performance of baccalaureate nursing graduates on licensure examination. *Journal of Professional Nursing, 8*(6), 342–350

Rollant, P. (1983). *Test-taking tips. Self published handout.* Newnan, GA: Multi-Resources, Inc.

Rollant, P. (1988). Test-taking strategies for the NCLEX®-RN exam. *Imprint: The National Student Nurse Association Journal, 30*(3), 15–17.

Rollant, P. (1999). *Soar to success: Do your best on nursing tests.* St. Louis: Elsevier.

Rollant, P. (2006). *2006 Content and test-taking skills for NCLEX®.* Navarre, FL: Author.

Seldomridge, L. A., & DiBartolo, M. (2004). Can success and failure be predicted for baccalaureate graduates on the computerized NCLEX-RN? *Journal of Professional Nursing, 20*(6), 361–368.

Spielberger, C. D., & Associates. (1990). *Test attitude inventory.* Retrieved March 3, 2006, from http://www.mindgarden.com/products/tsans.htm

Waterhouse, J., Bucher, L., & Beeman, P. (1994). Predicting NCLEX-RN performance: Cross-validating an identified classification procedure. *Journal of Professional Nursing, 10*(4), 255–260.

Weinstein, C. E., Schulte, A. C, & Palmer, D. R. (1990). *The college version of LASSI.* Retrieved March 3, 2006, from http://www.hhpublishing.com/_assessments/LASSI/scales.html

Wood, R. M. (2005). Student computer competence and the NCLEX-RN examination: Strategies for success. *CIN: Computers, Informatics, Nursing, 23*, 241–243.

Yin, T., & Burger, C. (2003). Predictors of NCLEX-RN success of associate degree nursing graduates. *Nurse Educator, 28*(5), 232–236.

Index

Contents of Volume 1

Contents of Volume 2

Contents of Volume 3

Contents of Volume 4

SPRINGER PUBLISHING COMPANY

Teaching Cultural Competence in Nursing and Health Care

Marianne R. Jeffreys, EdD, RN

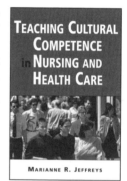

Preparing nurses and other health professionals to provide quality health care amid the increasingly multicultural and global society of the 21st century requires a new, comprehensive approach that emphasizes cultural competence education throughout professional education and professional practice. Written in response to this need, *Teaching Cultural Competence in Nursing and Health Care* is intended as a primary resource for educators and graduate students in academic settings, health care institutions, and professional associations.

It is the only book that presents a research-supported conceptual model and a valid, reliable corresponding questionnaire to guide educational strategy design, implementation, and evaluation. *Teaching Cultural Competence* provides readers with valuable tools and strategies for cultural competence education that can easily be adapted by educators at all levels.

Unique features of this book include:

- A model to guide cultural competence education

- A questionnaire for measuring and evaluating learning

- A guide for identifying at-risk individuals and avoiding pitfalls

- A wide selection of educational activities

- Techniques for diverse learners

- Vignettes, case examples, illustrations, tables, and assessment tools

2006 · 232pp · softcover · 0-8261-7764-6

11 West 42nd Street, New York, NY 10036-8002 • Fax: 212-941-7842
Order Toll-Free: 877-687-7476 • Order On-line: www.springerpub.com

Clinical Care Classification (CCC) System Manual

A Guide to Nursing Documentation

Virginia K. Saba, EdD, RN, FAAN, FACMI, LL

The Preeminent Nursing Terminology Classification System

"ABC Coding Solutions-Alternative Link developed ABC codes for nursing in collaboration with Dr. Virginia Saba, developer of the CCC system. Approximately two hundred ABC codes were developed from the CCC System of Nursing Interventions, to accurately document nursing and integrative health care processes, classify and track clinical care, and develop evidence-based practice models, thus filling significant gaps in older medical code sets."

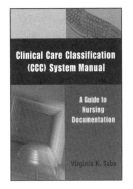

Clinical Care Classification (CCC) System Manual

A Guide to Nursing Documentation

Virginia K. Saba

—**Connie Koshewa,** Practitioner Relations Director
ABC Coding Solutions-Alternative Link

"The International Classification for Nursing Practice (ICNP®) is a program of the International Council of Nurses (ICN). One of the first steps in the development of the ICNP® was to collect and compare all the nursing concepts in existing nursing terminologies, including the CCC. To facilitate the goal of ICNP® as a unified nursing language system, a project is underway to map the CCC to the ICNP® Version 1.0. This work will facilitate evaluation and ongoing development of both terminologies and allow ICN to compare data using CCC codes with data from other standard nursing terminologies.

—**Amy Coenen,** PhD, RN, FAAN, Director
ICNP® Program, International Council of Nurses

2006 · 280 pp · softcover · 0-8261-0268-9

11 West 42nd Street, New York, NY 10036-8002 • Fax: 212-941-7842
Order Toll-Free: 877-687-7476 • Order On-line: www.springerpub.com

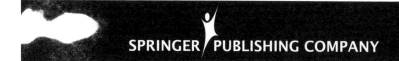

SPRINGER / PUBLISHING COMPANY

Teaching Evidence-Based Practice in Nursing

Rona F. Levin, PhD, RN
Harriet R. Feldman, PhD, RN, FAAN, Editors

"In their outstanding book, Rona Levin and Harriet Feldman...capture creative approaches to teaching evidence-based practice. This book includes comprehensive and unique strategies for teaching evidence-based practice for all types of learners across a variety of educational and clinical practice settings. The concrete examples of teaching assignments provided in the book bring the content alive and serve as a useful, detailed guide for how to incorporate this material into meaningful exercises for learners. Levin and Feldman's book is a truly wonderful, necessary resource for educators working in all healthcare professional programs as well as clinical settings." —From the Foreword by

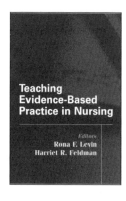

Bernadette Mazurek Melnyk, PhD, RN, CPNP/NPP, FAAN, FNAP

Based on the idea that nursing students and nurses at all levels can contribute to the development of a scientific base for nursing practice by critiquing and questioning guidelines, treatments, and outcomes of their own practice, this book examines the ways in which the teaching and learning of evidence-based practice (EBP) occurs. The book provides useful strategies for educators and facilitates the work of faculty to develop curricula that incorporate EBP and the work of nurses implementing EBP in the clinical setting.

Partial Contents

Part I: Setting the Stage

Part II: The Basics of Teaching/Learning Evidence-Based Practice

Part III: Teaching/Learning Evidence-Based Practice in the Academic Setting

Part IV: Teaching/Learning Evidence-Based Practice in the Clinical Setting

2006 · 400pp · softcover · 0-8261-3155-7

11 West 42nd Street, New York, NY 10036-8002 • Fax: 212-941-7842
Order Toll-Free: 877-687-7476 • Order On-line: www.springerpub.com

Notes